ABOUT THE AUTHOR

Colin was born and raised in Kettering, where he attended the local Grammar School. After a compelling call to the ministry, he studied at London Bible College (now London School of Theology) where he gained a London University Bachelor of Divinity honours degree. Colin served five churches during his 42 years in ministry.

In 2001 he was diagnosed with Parkinson's disease, but was able to continue to work until his retirement in 2012. He has been married for over 50 years and has three sons and seven grandchildren.

To my wonderful wife Wendy.

Colin Edmondson

SONGS
THROUGH
THE NIGHT

AUSTIN MACAULEY PUBLISHERS™

LONDON • CAMBRIDGE • NEW YORK • SHARJAH

A CIP catalogue record for this title is available from the British Library.

ISBN 9781398436138 (Paperback)
ISBN 9781398436145 (ePub e-book)

www.austinmacauley.com

First Published 2022
Austin Macaulay Publishers Ltd
1 Canada Square
Canary Wharf
London E14 5AA

ACKNOWLEDGEMENTS

My thanks to those who encouraged me to write this book, and to those who checked my spelling and grammar.

CHAPTERS

FOREWORD

This book is about a journey, a moving, fascinating journey in the face of great adversity. In 2001, Colin Edmondson began three years of progressive physical decline with Parkinson's disease. Colin takes us into the many and complex issues when faced with a life-changing diagnosis, from who needs to know to the burden of informing others. Then the many different and conflicting responses to this devastating news, often leading to a profound sense of isolation and sometimes hurt.

After receiving prayer for his healing, Colin experienced a significant period of stability and indeed improvement in his condition, which enabled him to complete the race before him as a Christian minister. With restored strength and freedom from the distressing symptoms of his illness he was also able, in the company of his wife Wendy, to return to his love of walking in the Highlands of Scotland, something which he thought he would never do again.

Colin writes about his experience, both the highs and lows, with his strikingly wonderful gift for words. He is an accomplished writer of Christian poems, and the reader will be stirred by Colin's ability to express his deepest experiences in language both sublime and evocative. This book is written by one whose eyes are fixed on Jesus, the initiator and goal of our faith. His stated purpose in this book is to share his love of Jesus with the desire that others should come to experience his healing love. To this end, he draws on stories of suffering and illness in the Bible and explains why these are still relevant for us today.

For Colin, the years when life returned to normal were not to last forever. So, what can be learned from this? Was Colin not healed after all? If he was, why did the disease return? If it is God's will that certain people bear these heavy crosses, there will be good reasons for this: for those who carry this cross as well as for those who watch from afar or who share the journey with words and deeds of comfort and support. Twenty years after his diagnosis, he is still in a better place than immediately before he experienced God's healing in 2003.

A major contribution of this book is that it calls for the sufferer to be seen and known for who they really are, each with their unique identity as a person. Awareness of this basic human need is paramount in both the pastoral and medical professions.

Colin's story will resonate with those fellow sufferers from this debilitating disease, and their loved ones and companions, on this long journey; I also suspect that it will make connections with many who live with other serious chronic illnesses. There are no easy days, just those which are perhaps less difficult. Every day demands courage and faith that all is not lost. Adjustments are necessary, but life is still worth living.

Apart from writing inspirational poems, Colin has provided us with this volume, drawn from a rich seam of Christian experience. It is clear to me that his suffering has not diminished his joy in family life, or his desire to grow in his relationship with God. These reflections are shared knowing that there are others on the same or similar journeys. In *Songs through the Night*, we will witness great courage and honesty, in a story so movingly told. I am confident it will give courage and bring hope to other travellers along this dark and often lonely road.

Dr John Dyer, Birchington, 18 July 2021

INTRODUCTION

This book was written with the desire to bring blessing and encouragement to those who suffer. At the same time, I wish to bring understanding to those who care for the suffering. It is written not as a philosophical apologetic but as an attempt to chart a way through it. I write as a Christian pastor for well over forty years, as a preacher/teacher of over 50 years, as having a BD (Hons), twice a part-time hospital chaplain and finally one who has battled with Parkinson's for over nineteen years.

These reflections began to be written when first diagnosed with Parkinson's disease. The original title was *Songs in the Night*, and the reasons for the change to '*through the Night*' will become obvious as the story unfolds. What is recorded is my response at the time. The parts in italics were recorded at or close to the events they relate. I hope this and the personal nature of the account is a help and not a hindrance to understanding. This comes not as an academic study divorced from life but as something forged by the fires of life's realities. My desire is to encourage and promote in some small way the ministering of Christ's love to needy people. If understanding and compassion are brought to others and the healing love of Christ extended in any way, it will have done what was intended.

I have reason to thank many people. Those who pray for me, without whom I doubt I would have survived the trial. My churches during this time, for their kindness, care and patience with an ailing pastor. Above all my wife Wendy who cared so constantly in my trials for me and never once made me think it was a burden to her. She is God's greatest blessing to me on earth.

The story that will unfold is one of amazing love and mercy from God to a very ordinary man. My prayer is that you will know that love too.

When the earth quakes & the mountains fall –

Psalm 46:

God is our shelter and strength,
always ready to help in times of trouble.
So we will not be afraid, even if the earth is shaken
and mountains fall into the ocean depths;
even if the seas roar and rage,
and the hills are shaken by the violence.
The LORD Almighty is with us;
the God of Jacob is our refuge.

Chapter 1

SONGS FOR THE NIGHT OF TEARS

Facing the Reality

'Yesterday, the 12 February 2001, a slow fuse was lit on the rest of my life. It came in a brisk no-nonsense statement "You have Parkinson's disease". Of course, it was already there, but now sentence was pronounced and I knew my likely end. I knew it was true for me as for everyone else that one day I will face the last enemy, death. But it was anonymous, and the time indefinite. Now it has a face and I have a probable time period; I have a decade before major disability is likely to strike and then decline until one day I choke or fall. Suddenly the ending of my life is defined. It is similar to the time I stood before my father's grave and saw the ending of my youth. Now I begin the last part of my life and I will carry this uninvited companion with me all the way. In the Bible story, Jacob wrestled with God for just one night, I will wrestle and fight this one enemy the rest of my days.

I was quite objective at first and in control, pleased with myself that I could make firm and sensible decisions about treatment. But we vowed not to hide feelings – the time left to us is too precious to use in any other way than with honesty and openness. I have sat alongside too many struggling in isolation with the pain of suffering to pretend. The rest of the journey must be clear and pure. We talked about *how we needed to respond, how we felt, and we renewed commitments to each other. We talked for some time, because it is 'we', my sweet companion and I, who will tread this journey together. I didn't want to burden her with this, always wanted to bring her joy, but now we face a greater challenge than Suilven* together and at the last it will win the day.*

This afternoon it finally hit me – the enormity, the final degrading awfulness. The sorrow claimed me as I was rehearsing in my mind what I would say to my three sons, how I would reassure them, and what their reactions might be and having to admit, to explain, that one day it would take hold of me. Whatever the delay, this thing will finally put its ropes around me, degrade me and cause my end. So I collapsed and howled and wept and knew my enemy. But I can still rob it of victory. It can claim my body but not my spirit.

I don't want to tell the boys. I must and it must be me, but I don't want to tell them. I don't want to cause them pain.'

Sooner or later pain, suffering, is a challenge we all face and we all wish we didn't. I wrote the above in a cloud of tears the day after the diagnosis was given. I was fifty-three and yet termed '*young* Parkinson sufferer'!

That first day, Monday February 12th, after we heard the news and I had my blood tests taken, we went home to hug each other and weep in each other's arms. It was a day of occasional tears and constant returning to Parkinson's, scratching round it a little like a new scab that had formed over a recent wound. When it itched for attention we scratched at it gently and briefly. Although I had mild 'flu as well, I eventually dosed myself up and we went to the London Museum and got ourselves two tickets to a concert by James Galway at the Barbican. So that evening we floated off into mystic musical rapture and for a few

---

*   Suilven is a precipitously steep and somewhat famous mountain in Scotland that we had climbed together the previous year.

moments forgot about incurable diseases. Yet from time to time it would drift into consciousness. It was, I think, a statement of faith, an affirmation of life, that the future still holds good times.

We continued like this the following day until I was left alone on that Tuesday afternoon. The power of the emotions hit me so unexpectedly, and yet necessarily, I believe. As I mentally reviewed how I would break the news to my children, mental pictures of my mother, who also suffered Parkinson's, rushed into my mind. Her body bent forward, little tottering steps, drooling from the mouth, hands trembling so much that she could hardly carry anything, and a voice so quiet that it was hard to distinguish a word even when I bent down to put my ear near her. And this was to be my future too. However long it would take, it would get me in the end, I felt. I can write this now dispassionately, but at the time the grief broke through me like a tidal wave.

Kind people tried to reassure me. 'The drugs today are so much better than they used to be'. They are, but eventually their effectiveness wears off. The end result doesn't change, I thought. 'We are only five/ten years from a cure.' But ignorance of the cause or causes of Parkinson's still remains. False dawns abound, and we will only know we have a cure when it has happened. The intention is to keep you from despair, to try to keep you from the depression that often grips Parkinson sufferers, and to encourage a 'positive mental attitude'. All this seems commendable, but for me the issue was first to look the beast squarely in the face. It might scare me to my finger ends but I didn't want any pretence, any running from reality, and no short cuts or avoidance strategies. So we trawled the web and found out what there was to be discovered about the illness and I saw my likely future. I wept and shouted and wondered how long I had to wait before this thing would rob me of my ministry.

There are those Christians who will be disappointed with the above account. They would tell me perhaps that

I am accepting a lie of Satan and that as a child of God I have a right to health. They would want this to be the reality I was affirming. I will speak later of other peoples' responses to my disability, including various Christian ones. As a Christian minister, I am particularly susceptible to these and to the target of other people's expectations. However, whatever the final outcome of faith and medical care, I think that some kind of 'facing the enemy' may be needed in cases of serious illness. People who have, for example, been diagnosed with brain tumours and malignant cancers have recounted to me their own kind of 'facing the enemy' and the grief that explodes from them when they have. This is no less necessary for other kinds of loss or trauma. I remember a woman telling me of the tragic moment when she stood with her husband beside the hospital bed of their dying teenage son. At the moment he died, her husband said without tear or tremor in his voice: *'The Lord gave and the Lord taketh away. Blessed be the name of the Lord.'* I am not sure what the effect was on the husband, as the lady was widowed before I knew her. I do know that she was emotionally crippled for years because she had never been allowed to grieve properly. I therefore think of this 'facing the enemy' and expressing grief as a healthy thing and it enabled me to make some positive steps forward from that watershed (literally!). The people who surround the sick or bereaved person need simply to understand and accept. I did not look for answers or instant healing, but those who would hear and stand with me and accept me with my limitations. My wife served as sounding board and sharer of my grief admirably, as did some of my friends.

Is this a biblical response? Does it come from faith or unbelief? Certainly, many Old Testament characters knew how to shout and complain to God, to weep and to sorrow. Famously, Jeremiah said:

'Cursed be the day I was born......why did I ever come out of the womb to see trouble and sorrow and to end my days in shame?' (Jeremiah 20:14,18.)

But are such expressions of pain right for New Testament believers who have so clear a hope and the empowering Spirit to comfort them? It is certainly a very human response and, remembering who created us, is that to be entirely despised? We have limited knowledge, often vivid imaginations, and only partial grasp of God's infinite wisdom. Is the alternative – a kind of beatific calm – the appropriate response to being told you have an incurable, progressive disease like Parkinson's or, say, a battle with cancer? There is *'a time to weep and a time to laugh'* says the writer of Ecclesiastes (3:4). The day of tears comes to us all and therefore needs to be accepted and offered up to God as much as any other life experience. Indeed, there are times when God calls us to shed tears and it would be inappropriate or even wrong not to. So, Isaiah (a prophet of God) tells the people of Israel that they are having a great party when they should have been crying before God. *'The Lord, the Lord Almighty, called you on that day to weep and to wail... but see there is joy and revelry'* (see the Bible book of Isaiah, chapter 22 verses 12,13). In danger, they decide they may as well just have a good time while they could. *'Till your dying day this sin will not be atoned for'* is the chilling judgement. The concern in Isaiah is for a people who have given up all hope when they should be turning back to God in repentance for the sin that brought them into the mess in the first place. They should be resting in the God Who could deliver them and will bring His covenant people into a place of blessing. They lacked faith and confidence in God. Shedding tears, expressions of grief can then come out of faith and confidence in God. Despite the pain and fears of the present and our uncertainties about the future, we are assured that our God has not abandoned us and is willing and able to bring us through.

Our confidence is in a God Who actually cares and enters into our sorrows. It is this God who can absorb our grief and transform it. The right place for tears is, then, before the God Whom we may barely sense and only glimpse through the shadows in the darkness of the hour. Yet this offering too we can bring – the broken heart, the hurt we feel. This too He will accept. At such times what counts is not how close we feel He is to us, but how near He actually is. I am reminded of a lady I know who loved spiders. When she saw them indoors she would tenderly cradle them in her hands and take them outside to safety. In the same way that God appears at times to us, she would be only a shadowy being to the spider and her care frightening. What mattered for them, though, was her readiness to cradle them in her hands and not stamp on them as most would do. Shadowy as His presence can seem at dark moments, He cradles us in His hands to bring us through to another place.

The outcome of such an offering of our pain or sorrow, shock or loss is also good. Verses 5 and 6 from Psalm 126 suggest that tears are not necessarily negative in their results *'for those who sow in tears will reap with songs of joy.'* The challenge to the sorrowing here is perhaps to keep sowing. I was reminded that God's purpose for my life did not stop because someone told me that I had an incurable disease. Ultimately it may rob me of my present ministry, but it will not rob me of ministry. That remains. In his book *To the Usual Suspects*, John Goldingay talks about his wife who suffers from MS. She ministers more powerfully to the people with whom she comes into contact than he ever could. 'I have this hunch that long after anything I have ever said about the Old Testament, about which I care passionately, has disappeared from most people's memories, some aspect of the memory of Anne abides with them [his students], and in some way they have been shaped by her, as I have been shaped and as my sons have' (p60). I believe this because I have seen such ministry over the years. My response, in my pain, was to commit myself to share the love of God in whatever way I am given strength and ability. That at least I can give. My tears will be accompanied by sowing the good news of Jesus. That is my desire.

Perhaps the most powerful example of crying over trials to come was in a garden called Gethsemane. It is at that point in Jesus' life when the cross is around the corner – the next day. He knows He will be crucified and He knows that all dignity will be stripped from Him, and that massive pain and a terrifying sense of abandonment by God awaits Him. In a matter of hours the process of humiliation and torture would begin. I find myself moved as I contemplate the thought that He too knew what it was to anticipate the degradation of His human dignity. Crucifixion was designed to do that, and so, ultimately, does Parkinson's. Jesus' response was, according to Hebrews 5:7, to offer up '*prayers and petitions with loud cries and tears.*' He was '*in anguish*' (Luke 22:44), '*overwhelmed with sorrow to the point of death*' (Mark 14:34 and Matthew 26:38) – all of which makes my grief a passing cloud. To compare my trials in any way with His is to feel almost ridiculous. His was so much weightier a sorrow, so much more significant and voluntary. There is nothing voluntary about my disease, it has been bestowed on me by causes as yet unknown. Nor do I imagine it to be on behalf of others, the way Jesus' suffering was. He was degraded and died to save others, to obtain my forgiveness and eternal life. Of course, this applies not just to me but to all that are ready to receive this new beginning from God. His loving act still cries out to us inviting us accept His life-changing gift. In response I can only say: 'Father forgive me, a sinner.'

Yet gloriously different as His suffering is, it also treads a path for us that some of us can identify with. He too broke out into cries and tears in facing up to suffering yet to be experienced. Is it because He shouted out that the human side of Jesus was able to face the actual suffering so calmly? That, and the submission to God. '*If it is possible, take this cup from me. Yet not as I will, but as You will.*' We must ever desire to be rid of the illness because it is an evil. There is something unhealthy about enjoying ill-health. By a 'good sickness' some obtain attention, perhaps? Or freedom from responsibility? For some, 'Do you want to be made well and be healed of your ailments?' is a relevant question. But finally, we need to submit to God's will in the confidence that whatever He wills for us is the best way to glorify Him. This is no wailing litany of defeat accepted, of resignation to whatever happens, but a war cry. By it we rise up in the situation in which we are placed and battle for the Lord. In this we bear fruit. Here, by some means, we extend the Kingdom of God. That is my faith for the future. The God Who has never failed me this last 70 years or so will not fail me now. So, the crying out to God that leads to abandonment to His will is surely right. To do so in the faith that He will work out His purpose in my life is not a matter of giving up. It is rather to look for another kind of victory, that which is won in, and through, my weakness. 'Your will be done' is not an excuse, but our greatest testament of faith.

One of my daughters-in-law is a fine example of this. All her life she has had to battle with a condition that causes constant pain and physical trials, as she can dislocate a joint or two at the shake of a hand or a jolt to her head. When driving her anywhere, you can no doubt imagine how hard we try to drive very, very smoothly, avoiding as many potholes as possible. Her condition requires her to wear a leg brace. She has a particularly well designed one. This leads strangers to come up to her and enquire about this piece of engineering excellence. Such encounters have a tendency to broaden and include such questions as 'How can you be so cheerful when you suffer as you do?' She then explains how her relationship with God makes all the difference. There is nothing pompous about it, but a caring sharing of the comfort and hope she has received through her faith in Jesus. Nor is it that we are saved from feeling the pain and loss. But when we sit alongside those who suffer as fellow sufferers, we can share mutual understanding in the fellowship of those in pain and loss. It is a thirsty man in a hot and arid desert uncovering a well of water for another dying of thirst. Do we have any right to tell someone battling with devastating illness or loss how they should feel? Does it help those battered by bodily ill-health or shocked by deep personal loss to have someone in easier circumstances demand that they should be responding some other way? My own experience is that it makes the sufferer feel even more isolated.

It may seem strange to belabour the point about the validity of tears and loud cries, but it arises from witnessing the struggles of those who fight back their emotions, imagining it as some kind of virtue. They are praised for their strength and courage. The social pressure, especially for men, is to stay collected and calm. The wartime slogan 'Keep calm & carry on' has widespread acceptance. 'Laugh and the whole world laughs with you, weep and you weep alone,' the saying goes. Who wants to be alone at such a time? So the pressure is on to cope acceptably and to truly weep alone. Those who follow this path are 'so brave' and highly commended, but they weep secretly into their pillows at night and their souls are seared by the fire and hardened against joy as well as pain. The burden is sometimes added to by well-meaning Christians who are looking for you to be so taken up by Christian hope that any tears are of joy not of pain. Perhaps there is a different way. Own up to the pain but release it to God. Let the tears be healing tears as you look up to a divine love that has the future in His hands.

Nonetheless, anything can be overdone. **There is no virtue in living in the valley of tears all the time.** After Gethsemane, Jesus faced the cross with great courage and few tears. The way seems to be to bring it to God in as much faith as you have and not just rely on the tears for emotional release. The Bible heroes addressed very bold complaints to God that expressed graphically just how they felt. Rarely, though, is this the end of the story. After pouring out their hearts they turn to some kind of thanksgiving or expression of future hope. For this reason, my song for the night of tears is Psalm 42:1-5 which climaxes in the Psalmist talking to himself.

'Why are you downcast, O my soul? Why so disturbed within me? Put your hope in God, for I will yet praise him, my Saviour and my God.'

Perhaps tears can be a self-indulgence too, at times. Perhaps we do have a need to talk to ourselves and remember before God that this sorrow too will pass. For the Christian there is always a future and a hope and eventually we need to focus on this. Having passed through the valley of tears, as we must, we look up into the face of our Father and find it has become the highway to hope. Without cutting short the time of sorrowing, there is a time too to refocus away from the loss and on to the hope.

As for those around the sufferer, the call is perhaps to '*mourn with those who mourn*'. Often, people struggle to know how to approach those who have experienced some tragedy or other. Not infrequently, they avoid them. They try to explain their fears with words like: 'I wouldn't know what to say.' Meanwhile, the sufferer is made to feel like the proverbial leper or that they have some highly contagious disease. I have been told by suffering people that folk they know well literally cross over to the other side of the road to avoid them. They are abandoned to their grief, and the isolation increases. What lies behind this reluctance to engage or even chat with those who are experiencing trials? Do those who do this imagine themselves saying something hurtful and so add to their pains? Is it that they think they may do more harm than good? Or is it too near their own fears they are afraid to face? Is it about **our** discomfort rather than **their** need? Yet the road to depression is to bottle things up, wanting 'to be strong' out of pride or because there is no one who will listen and just accept whatever you feel. Lonely isolation can be a killer. In 2020 nearly every country in the world felt the impact of isolation when under lockdown rules. The intention was to try to restrain Covid-19. Although we had connections through the internet, it proved to be a time of real trial.

Perhaps we are hurting for a friend or relative as we recognise the trial they face. As we sit with those who suffer, or think of them, we can more readily identify with their distress and make all the more potent our prayers. We join with them, and our cries to God mingle with theirs. Jesus looked for companions in His night of sorrow and found them asleep to His need. Perhaps we have all too often repeated the mistake. Instead of 'weeping with those who weep', the temptation is there to point to the good too early in the process. In our desire to comfort and lessen the trial or shorten its impact, we offer some 'pain-killer' or even false hope. But these don't heal; they numb us to the hurt. Sometimes the words of supposed hope only serve to isolate the one going through the difficulty. Their feelings are not being heard. It is amazing to me that the Bible story of Job, who suffered repeated tragedy, has his friends sitting with him silently for seven days. It was still not long enough.

Eventually I came to write the words that follow as my own response to my condition – but it came sometime later.

'… into your hands'

If it were possible I would avoid
This trial of constant suffering
That persists in further humbling
Me. This path is not by choice.

First I face the pain
The stab of my body hurting
Throwing out its harsh warning
Like an alarm screaming for attention.

SONGS FOR THE NIGHT OF TEARS

Then the sense of loss in limitation
That makes me old before age can,
Longing still for the easy freedom
That fitness casually gave by donation.

Then I am touched by suffering,
The interpretation of pain, that makes
The heart revolt at the indignities
So that the inner self frustrated shakes.

When then I come to this place
Where by choice you bore the loss,
The pain of torture and a cross
I gaze astonished at this grace.

For me you chose the path of pain
For me the trials taken and the shame.
Like me, if possible, you would have avoided
This humiliating suffering upon you loaded.

Yet it was too big a price to pay
To face our loss and avoid the cross.
Thus love is measured by the cost
And then paid to retrieve the lost.

Gently I come in my pains and kneel
Wishing and praying that you might heal.
But a deeper wonder comes to light
Your presence makes my weakness might.

Here I look up into your face
And know that we travel together
The trails of trials. Here I discover
Not only comfort but blessings of grace.

I learn then as I watch
Your patience as You endure
And yield up Your spirit at the last.
So I yield mine and all on you I cast.

'Father, into your hands I yield my spirit...'

Chapter 2

LEARNING TO SING IN A STRANGE PLACE

Adjusting to 'Incurable Disease'

I have been asked if I expected the diagnosis. During the previous three years I had developed symptoms that crept up on me so slowly that I was hardly aware of them. Yet I increasingly knew something was wrong and, I feared, seriously wrong. My favourite self-diagnosis was that I had suffered some kind of minor stroke as my right arm seemed stiff and like a clumsy lump. My handwriting and keyboard skills were deteriorating and my energy levels dropping. All this whilst adjusting to the frenetic pace of London after over 12 years serving in the comparative calm of the New Forest. Furthermore, I was serving as senior minister in a very demanding church that was full of very gifted people and had high expectations of me, its minister. We called it a *'house of prayer for all nations'* (*Matthew* 21:13). This it truly was, with 30 or more different nationalities. With this mix of nationalities was added people of every strata of society, active members of all three political parties and plenty of people with decided opinions. It made for a very lively church. Challenging enough when I was ill; how would I be up to the task with Parkinson's? Five-year action plans and careful management systems would have gone down a treat. Even when not afflicted with Parkinson's disease, this conflicted with my free-wheeling personality. My main and abiding passion is a deepening spirituality based on a personal relationship with God through the constantly astonishing person of Jesus Christ. This is brought to life through the Holy Spirit. These things are not words to me but root into the depths of my being and experience. I am constantly amazed by this, somewhat in the way that I am surprised at the extent of my wife's love. I stumble along, trailing Jesus at distance, and every now and again He stops and He grabs hold of me and hugs me. I know that I am an awkward customer but He doesn't seem to mind.

I like to share all this with others. I am not one for big organisation, but for progressing in this simple but profoundly challenging stuff of loving God and each other. This seems to me more revolutionary than the Internet. Thus, I was increasingly under pressure from a church, some of whom wanted me to be someone else (but a different 'someone else' according to their particular pref-erence) and at the same time I found my ability to respond to the situation diminishing. Having come from a church where I was respected at least, it was a novel experience. I was fortified by the knowledge that the God who had used us to unite and build up churches in the past would not fail us now. It was hard going. There were one or two who were unforgiving of my weaknesses and left. In many ways this pain was greater than my illness. Some I had thought to be mature Christians could only see as far as the 'performance' on Sunday, etc. They perhaps sought for a church that was a kind of spiritual filling station where they could top up for the 'real action' elsewhere. They considered me unable to deliver and so went to some well-known London centre of whatever it was they thought they wanted. I wasn't looking for excuses. I never could do this ministry thing anyway. I learnt years ago that if anything was to happen, God had to do it. Nearly all my ministerial colleagues are better than I am at the professional things. I learnt that it was God or nothing. I merely had that reinforced.

God always humbles you more than you think is really necessary. It seems I still had some way to go. So I battled through, took what criticisms there were and any angry letters, and placed the odd card of thanks or encouragement on the mantelpiece in my study and covered up or compensated for my increasing clumsiness and weariness. Those critics were far from being many and I was to find a number of amazingly supportive and caring people too.

Those four words 'You have Parkinson's disease' therefore came like lightning from the sky. I did not expect this at all. I am not alone in experiencing this kind of shock. Others too, even knowing that they are somehow ill, don't really suspect the reality of some terrible diagnosis. Even if they do suspect, the confirmation of their fears can be just as shocking and disturbing. In my case the neurologist gave me some words that I held on to – 'You should be able to work for some years yet. I think you have a slow-developing variety.' I appreciated the caring approach of the consultant neurologists at King's College Hospital, London, and their readiness to answer my questions. But do medical staffs realise what a bombshell they let fall with such simple words and how vital the words they use next? I give the folk whom I consulted full marks. For me no hedging or cover up would do. I wanted the simple realities. If that had not been given me then would I trust their other comments and reassurances? I seriously doubt it.

The next few months were made up of a cycle of adjustments and sharing my news with an ever-growing circle of people. It is a process that all in similar situations must go through. Ministerial life has the added dimension of being lived at a very public level. People examine you with studious care. This is not unnatural, as they want to know whether the things you say and represent are real to you or not. For this reason, integrity and a consistent personal spiritual life are vital ingredients of Christian leadership. It is not the kind of public life that a leading politician or media celebrity has to live out, but it is public nevertheless. Within this, judgements too abound. So the sharing of this news will also be subject to scrutiny. Christian friends and acquaintances can also be the most supportive people around as I have observed. This background is necessary to understand the context of my life for the months following that diagnosis.

First, there was the emotional adjustment. The tears came freely at first and I had moments when unexpectedly something on TV or something someone said hit an emotional chord and I was fighting back the flow. Bit by bit this initial turbulence and the sense of treading on fragile ground subsided. After five months I felt that life was fairly much back to normal emotionally. But acceptance and adjustment, I have found, is a constant exercise. With fluctuating periods of good and bad days, you just think things are stabilised and you are more capable again when a bad time comes and you struggle to come to terms with your incapacity. A progressive disease means constantly coming to terms with a new loss. The initial shock may pass; the challenge does not. At first, the crisis threw me close to God. I had to depend on Him. Later, the loss of energy restricted my time in prayer and reflection. New patterns of life needed to be established so that a greater loss was not sustained. The one thing I wanted to be left with was my relationship with God.

Secondly, I had to let others know and break the news. This meant repeatedly having to face up to the issue. This in itself was no easy task. I had to accept, absorb and respond to the feelings and responses of others. Yet keeping it secret was not an option. It would mean denying my true self and the openness of real fellowship that I have taught. Each Parkinson sufferer I suppose will decide their own policy on this according to their personality and situation. Again, this is true for anyone having to communicate some great loss. Those around them need to understand the extra pressure disclosure brings for anyone who has to share bad news.

Thirdly, I had to learn to continue working even though preoccupied with my illness. Inside I cried out for a few months' Sabbatical so that I could come to terms with things and think of the implications for my future. But Wendy was still working and anyway this was not on offer. It was probably a mercy too. Perhaps real acclimatisation needs to be done in the context of ordinary, everyday duties. Strangely, at the same time we faced a whole stream of trying practical problems that were not of our making: for example, a burst water pipe whose repair entailed the demolition of a large gate post and part of our front wall and took endless negotiation to get the job done. Nevertheless, at times the best I could do in my work was to try to survive. In working through the implications of this new situation I found I had little energy left for working at exciting new visions for the church. Had I a 9-7 job, I can only imagine the sheer collapse that would come at the end of the day. How hard that would be for the rest of the family.

Fourthly, I had to deal with the impact on those close to me. The truth is those around us have to make adjustments and face loss too. Though not as severe as the death of a partner, the sense of loss has features common to bereavement. Kubler-Ross famously wrote of the five stages of grief. These stages are said to be experienced in the order of:

1. Denial
2. Anger
3. Bargaining
4. Depression
5. Acceptance

However, my experience of caring for people soon showed me that you cannot be so prescriptive about people's journey through grief. Perhaps the closer the relationship, the greater the impact will be. A wife or husband has to face the prospect of an ever-changing situation. The once strong and capable partner is not what they were and furthermore is different day to day. When these things strike they don't just strike the individual but a whole circle of others. The quality of our relationships will then determine our ability to support one another. The loss of real community has, perhaps, raised the necessity of the 'support group'. My gratitude is ever towards my chief 'supporter', Wendy – now my wife of over 49 years – who treats me with endless patience and understanding even on my worst days. Such blessings are priceless. We have made it a rule to share what is happening openly with each other. This means we are less likely to misunder-stand each other as well as just simply being together in it.

I have observed many couples handling the difficulties or tragedies of life and not meeting them *together*. Some-times they co-habit the same area of sorrow but deal with it separately. For example, some time ago I visited a family annually on the anniversary of a daughter's death. At the beginning I held four totally different conversations at once as each shared their grief. Father, mother and siblings were all locked into their own sorrows and were not sharing each other's or dealing with it collectively. My family didn't want to make this mistake. Furthermore, to leave each other to guess what the other one was feeling would have been making unfair demands. We didn't want to set each other complex puzzles to work out, but instead help each other to simply understand. The words 'He/she should know without me telling him/her' are a common cause of communication breakdown and loss of closeness in relationship. When someone close knows 'something is wrong' but is left in the dark, they are given anxiety and, in addition, the feeling of rejection by being excluded. To share these things together gave us not only the oppor-tunity of drawing strength from one another, but also helped us to grow closer still, even in the trial. The bonds we establish as couples are not just strengthened by the joys we share but the sorrows we bear together. Some, sadly, let tragedy isolate them from each other – some-times to the extent of tearing them apart.

Perhaps the way it affected others, especially Wendy, was the hardest trial of all. If I had been the only one restricted by this disease it would have been easier. To know that your illness also robs the one dearest to you is harder to bear. I began to understand what elderly folk mean when they say: 'I don't want to be a burden to anyone.' When the desire of your heart is to bring joy and blessing to others, it is painful to think that you add to the difficulties of the people you love. Yet there can be a special kind of closeness in sharing times of trial if they are not resented. New depths of companionship can be discovered that compensate for all that you go through together.

It strikes me that the breakdown of marriage and family, the lack of deep relationships, is a threat to all those who face crises in life. Good as support groups often are, they are not open 24 hours and need does not surface according to timetable. I fear for the many lonely people facing these kinds of trials, and worse, who have no one close by their side. Perhaps there is mercy in God's way of doing things that we ignore to our own harm.

I close this chapter by saying that there are far worse things to face than Parkinson's disease. It is, after all, not immediately life-threatening but lifestyle-threatening. The challenge in the lives of many is far greater than I have described here. Yet as I track through my own struggles, I see some lines of correspondence between their experience and this chronicle. I write in the hopes that others may perhaps be helped a little or others come to understanding. But I believe that each person must be given the room to respond in their own way to their particular situation. People are not so 'programmed' that they respond in prescribed fashions. There is peculiar uniqueness about each human being, which is both their glory and the challenge for all who would support and cherish them. That challenge is to listen, to share and to care, whatever the manner of their dealing with it. But for me there was a song in this night of my tears.

'Blessed are those who weep now for they shall be comforted.'

Psalm 42:1–5

As a deer longs for a stream of cool water,
so I long for you, O God.
I thirst for you, the living God;
when can I go and worship in your presence?
Day and night I cry,
and tears are my only food;
all the time my enemies ask me,
'Where is your God?'
My heart breaks when I remember the past,
when I went with the crowds to the house of God
and led them as they walked along,
a happy crowd, singing and shouting praise to God.
Why am I so sad?
Why am I so troubled?
I will put my hope in God,
and once again I will praise him,
my Saviour and my God.*

---

* American Bible Society. (1992). The Holy Bible: The Good news Translation (2nd ed., Ps 42:1–5). New York: American Bible Society.

Chapter 3

SONGS COMPOSED BY COMMUNITIES OF CARE

Facing Others in The Night

The group that gathered around me were insistent and definite about their demands – they wanted me healed and **now**. Compassionate, but lacking real understanding of my condition, they laid hands on me and insisted that I should be made well. 'Use your right hand to write something,' said one, looking for an instant miracle. 'Do not accept the lies of the devil,' said another. All of them were church leaders and all of them believed I should be healed, some that it was in the covenant that God had made with me as a child of God. Some claimed I had the right to good health. This was the reaction of just one of the groups to which I related.

Most of us have circles of people we are involved with at some level or another. They may only intersect through you. The fashionable word is to term them 'networks', using the model of electrical circuits that connect with each other. For Christians, the connections should run deeper than casual contact and, at their best, nowhere does a person receive more care in time of need than in a church community. It doesn't always work out that way, of course; church folk are only trainee saints and sometimes get things terribly wrong. Sometimes they are not Christ's folk at all, or have forgotten that they are, and miss the main thing in spite of everything they hear and witness. Yet my experience was that most showed a level of care. They wanted the best for me. Whatever the problems I encountered, genuine concern was at the heart of the majority of people's responses. For that I am truly grateful and I hope I showed it. So I call this chapter 'Communities of Care' because that is what they are. Although they all cared, they were not all equally helpful and the levels of engagement were very different. In commenting on these very different responses in others, I wish only to share how that was experienced by me the sufferer, so that perhaps a little light is shed on the situation. If, as a result, some other person is the better supported and finds deeper understanding then I will have succeeded. In the process I would like to ask some questions about our understanding of divine healing.

One of the first hurdles for the newly diagnosed person is the business of simply telling others – as I have already mentioned. This is a series of emotional barriers that has to be somehow got through. At first, I found myself walking through a minefield of explosive feelings. I don't mean I collapsed into tears every time I told someone. I am a man after all, and men, on the whole, aren't supposed to do that sort of thing! But it was draining and exhausting and privately I had to manage the grief all over again. Furthermore, I was constantly surprised by my own responses. Different issues were involved in each case. I was conscious that for my family there was a threat in my news. I needed to reassure them that the disease is not simply genetic. Both my mother and my mother's sister suffered from Parkinson's, so the situation looked bad. Yet my three elder brothers are mercifully free of the disease and I know of no other cases within the family. At worst, there is an inherited tendency but not a direct genetic cause. (By the same token those Christians who might be tempted to look for some 'inter-generational curse' are unable to make a case for similar reasons. An 'inter-generational curse' is a concept that some evil/

curse is passed down through the generations.) So I had not only to share my news but to explain all this at the same time.

That first round was not easy, but necessary and strangely therapeutic. **Sometimes I wondered if I had heard correctly** and that the words had not been uttered by the neurologist and I didn't have Parkinson's disease after all. Once more I was grateful that Wendy had been there and I had a witness I could rely on. Yet it was good to talk about it. At different times the word was dropped into different 'pools' of people and I observed and absorbed the ripple of responses. I was linked to several different ministers' groups and I began with the 'safest' in terms of how I believed they would take the news. I also shared the news with my church leaders who were shocked enough to be uncharacteristically quiet. Eventually I stood before the church and told them too. They gathered around and with great fervour and differing convictions they laid hands upon me and prayed for me. Some prayed for my strength and help in the situation and others my deliverance from the disease.

Some may ask why I told the church before I absolutely had to. I think it is because I try to be honest and avoid pretence in my dealings with others. I felt that if I was to face people with any kind of integrity or humanity, I needed to share with them. I also owed it to them to let them know what I was battling with as I tried to minister. It might, after all, affect my ministry amongst them. At the same time I recognised that to do so was risky. After all who knew what their attitude might be? As I have already said, as a minister you face the trial of other peoples' expectations and convictions. They want you to be heroic and faith-filled and clearly triumphant. Do they want you to be as weak and vulnerable as they are? For some, the triumph they wanted was for me to pronounce confidence in my healing and to see it take place.

I am always moved when people, hearing of my condition, pray for me. Sometimes the prayer was offered by large gatherings. Perhaps the most dramatic was at a large missions meeting in southern Brazil in June 2003. Some of my leaders and myself had the opportunity to link up with the churches of Criciuma. Our purpose was to encourage each other, especially in terms of mission. So it was that we flew to the deep south of Brazil, to be alongside our new friends and for me to speak at a Missions Conference. Christians from a wide area, including Argentina, gathered in the city hall, which just about seated 1,000 or so generally young and enthusiastic Christians. When my turn came to speak, I included an apology if my voice did not carry as well as I would have wished, giving an explanation for this. After I had finished my apology, one of the Brazilian leaders suggested that they should pray for me. I knelt in the centre of the platform while the whole congregation erupted in prayer – very loud and very passionate prayer. Everybody prayed, all at once. This was for me! Or at least I think it was, but as they were all speaking in either Portuguese or Spanish, I didn't understand a word they said. It was a truly humbling experience. Although I was not physically totally restored, the warmth of their love and their respect strengthened the music of my soul.

With certain illnesses there is the risk of being somewhat diminished as a person in others' eyes. Wendy told me of a habit in one hospital, where she had been a nurse, of describing someone as, for example, 'a Parkinson', their identity being made into a disease. The danger was that people would see me as the minister who had Parkinson's disease and not as the person I am – for good or ill. I had seen this tendency to de-personalise or diminish the individual who has some ailment often enough in my times as a hospital chaplain to know it was a real issue. Yet I could not put on a show, and so the risk to reveal my condition was taken. For the church, the subtext was to know how far this would affect my work. The unsatisfactory answer was that I didn't really know, but for the time being nothing much should change. I could only promise to review things with them on a regular basis.

It should be mentioned that the problem of personal identity can affect the carers close to those who are seriously ill. There is the ever-present danger that they are seen only as the ailing person's nurse. For example, Gavin was widely known in the forest community where he lived. At 30-something he was confined to a wheelchair. His wife told me that on meeting up with people the only question they ever asked was 'How's Gavin?' She said her nightmare was that she would be knocked down in the High Street and someone would bend over her and ask 'How's Gavin?' Carers are people, too, with their own needs and issues. They suffer with the person who is ill.

Friends and churches where I had ministered previously had also to be included in this communication. It seemed like a long steeplechase that meant constantly jumping over the same hurdles. Mostly, with time and repetition, the emotional strain in doing this diminished. The whole process took months and was a trial within a trial. It is not surprising that some sufferers would rather avoid this altogether or find intermediaries to let people know. In the beginning it is like stabbing yourself repeatedly in the foot. It also means facing the uncertain passage of how they will react.

For the most part, the ministers I spoke to were not like the group I mentioned at the start of this chapter. They are, as a tribe, used to hearing other peoples' bad news and sympathising. Mostly they know how to ask questions and listen, rather than come up with simplistic 'answers' or even vague re-assurances. Most of my colleagues gave me a gentle and quiet hearing. Our area superintendent, the denominational leader who has the role of pastoring the pastors, gave very gentle and understanding support. She also enabled us to have a much-needed break. It was this gentle response that I felt was the most helpful. Somewhat unexpectedly, I found myself wanting to avoid any kind of high-powered healing service. I definitely didn't want people shouting and claiming things over me.

During this time, I visited a colleague suffering from a terminal cancer. We got talking about healing and he made the comment **that he believed in healing communities**. I was drawn to this idea of the caring community that, simply and quietly and with confidence, committed the sufferer to God. **I wanted to be placed in the healing stream that flows from God's presence.** I wanted to escape from anyone who might want to blast me with power. I think I instinctively feel that they are about self-promotion, not gospel proclamation – perhaps even 'fleecing the flock' for personal gain instead of caring and building them up in love. I am happy to say that such people are rare, but ever-ready, with false teaching or exaggeration (a form of lying), to exploit those in desperate need.

To return to the group I mentioned at the head of this chapter, I found the experience of the way they prayed for me strangely isolating. Part of the isolation was the feeling that they did not understand what it was I was facing or what I believed about it. I could have been suffering anything and the prayers would be the same. Furthermore, the words of encouragement took in no awareness of where I was in the situation. I realised how important it was to be heard and appreciated for who I was.

It is striking how Jesus dealt with the woman who had a haemorrhage. She came to Him in faith, but instead of shouting out like the blind man who Jesus met on another occasion, she simply stretched out her hand through the crush of the crowd and touched the edge of His coat. Although she was healed, this was not enough for Jesus. He stopped and enquired, 'Who touched me?' The disciples thought this was a little ridiculous considering the circumstances and said so. 'You see the people crowding against you,' they said, 'and yet you can ask who touched you?' However, Jesus persisted until the woman came forward, frightened as she was. Apparently, for Jesus, healing involved a very personal contact with Him. He wanted her to know that she counted as a person, that she mattered to him. Furthermore, He gave re-assurance and blessing. '*Daughter* [note the tenderness of the title], *your faith has healed you. Go in peace and be freed of your suffering.*' (Mark 5:24f.)

'Peace' communicated to Jesus' hearers something more than feeling calm and mellow. It also meant everything necessary to fulfil the life of peace. It meant having all the conditions necessary for not only being able to live in a state of harmony and tranquillity but also of enabling people to live to their full potential. It involved a combination of wholeness of spirit as well as material good and external security. For example, God's Kingdom of peace is set forward in Isaiah 32:15,16 thus:

'*Everywhere in the land righteousness and justice will be done. Because everyone will do what is right, there will be peace and security for ever. God's people will be free from worries and their homes peaceful and safe.*'

So, Jesus sought to bless the woman with more than physical well-being. When we give access only to physical good health, we are not completing the job. Jesus therefore ensured that the woman had personal contact with Him in order to bring her into a richer and fuller life altogether. In fact, the New Testament account of Jesus healing people shows us no formula applied in every case, but tailor-made interaction that varied according to the person's particular need, and the necessary means to give them the opportunity to discover the peace of God. We need then to ask, when we practise the ministry of healing, how well do we provide the opportunity for people to be dealt with individually? Is our approach flexible enough and does it enable people to access the peace of God? The practice of mass healings in public events seems to me a little impersonal and may be because the 'healer' focuses exclusively on 'giving glory to God' and imparting faith to others. People become then a kind of public trophy or a proof of divine activity in the world. This stems from an anxiety that perhaps God has abandoned us or is not around after all. So we demonstrate that He is here and ready to bless. This seems a worthy objective at first sight. If it comes from real faith there is some value, but if out of unbelief that is seeking assurance, less so perhaps.

Jesus naturally had no insecurity when He ministered, nor had He any need to 'prove God'. As a result, He wasn't afraid to deal with people privately, or take them round the corner out of sight of the crowd. He seemed more concerned with the individual and glorifying God by their wholeness. He also seemed less impressed over the kind of response to Him that was based on the spectacular miracle rather than on His words and deeds. This usually involved questions about their lives and some recognition of their beliefs.

I have one friend in particular who showed me this grace. He was the quickest to respond to the news of my diagnosis and travelled some miles to see me. Gerry didn't lecture me or seek to push his views about healing on to me, but brought a big box of goodies and listened to me express my heart. That was a healing moment for which I am so grateful. Sometimes we may be so eager to relieve the suffering that we can forget the sufferer.

This happened once or twice when visiting hospital, for example. Some time after the diagnosis, I began to have problems with voice production. I was referred, I was told, to one of the world's experts and found myself walking into the consulting room at a world-famous hospital unsure of what lay ahead. I am not accustomed to serious illness and so the whole thing was new to me even if hospitals are not. (I have served as part-time hospital chaplain.) I approached the smart-looking lady at the desk poring over my notes. I was aiming for an empty chair near her desk, but I was soon rounded up and they headed me off towards a machine whilst 'the expert' totally ignored me. I later wrote of this experience with tongue in cheek. The names have been changed.

Just another lesion

Only a visit to the therapist
'One of the best in the world,' she said.
So I waited without apprehension, 'last on the list'
He said. 'Colin Edmondson' at last, professionally read
And I was summoned into the lady lion's den.

There were three who presided:
A 'principal therapist' going grey and untidy,
A Frenchman observer mute and stationary,
And the chief, the queen of the piece, Miss Preston,
Who ignored me as she absorbed my notes
Which were clearly far more interesting than my person.

They talked briefly, briskly and with conviction
'The report was very thorough, but we will have an inspection.'
A piece of apparatus flanked my left,
The grey one sharply tried to keep my attention
As Miss Preston fiddled ominously with needles and kept
Preparing a long shining metal probe, deft
And businesslike but what will they attempt?

Then they attacked – 'Open your mouth,
Stick out your tongue, keep breathing,
Say E>E>E>E, while I thrust this thing
Deep into your buccal cavity.' 'Don't turn,
Or lower your chin, or close your mouth
Or stop breathing.
Just look at me and while
I hold your tongue we'll take pictures of your throat.'

Startled at this assault with no premeditation
Or the dignity of calm reflective explanation
I retched and gagged and couldn't see how
I could perform this trick of medical practice.
So they sprayed a local anaesthetic, said 'Swallow'
And numbed I performed the deed and nice

Clear pictures of my throat appeared on screen.

'There's your problem,' she said triumphantly. 'See
A cyst there and a lesion that we
Must investigate. The cyst we will remove
And investigate the other under general anaesthetic.
I will make an appointment for you to be admitted.'
There, it is said. A lesion, a named threat
And my first hospital stay and not just a visit.

I am not yet gripped by anxieties
But I can imagine lots of possibilities.
Cancer – benign or malignant.
Just another cyst or polyp or other ailment.
The future meets today and seems unsure,
But I need fear nothing or feel insecure
For He is the future come sickness or cure.

Yet I can't help but wonder –
Couldn't this team of great specialists
Meet me as a person and not one on their lists
Of clinical conundrums to ponder?
Gentleness, warmth, explanation, permission
Would perhaps have given some intimation
That I was human – and not just another lesion.

Christian or not, it is a lesson for all to absorb. There is more to an alcoholic than alcohol. There is more to the sick than sickness or disease. Healing is aided by recognising this and living it. One of the temptations of sickness is to let it define your life and absorb you. In refusing this, you can vote to live fully and constructively. The same leading consultant also said something to another doctor as I awaited that throat operation. As I lay on the trolley awaiting anaesthetic it was mentioned that I had Parkinson's. 'You can see it in the face,' she said, indicating that I had something of the Parkinson 'mask'. This is caused by the inability to 'tell' the face muscles to show expression.

As I frequently speak publicly as a part of my ministry, this is a challenging handicap. No one had even hinted that I exhibited this unfortunate symptom until then. She was very observant to notice this, but not necessarily wise in choosing that moment to broadcast it. It left me with a new issue to evaluate and deal with and no chance to talk it through with anyone for days. After the operation, I had to refrain from any talking at all for three days. After that I had to keep talk to a minimum for a week. This is quite a discipline for someone whose life revolves around speaking to others. Can you imagine having to keep all those helpful, witty and erudite comments to myself? No wonder I have since taken to writing.

These comments should not be taken as typical of all my experiences of medical people. Many have treated me with understanding and great kindness and are models of good practice. That someone at the top of her profession should make this kind of mistake indicates just how easily we fall into the trap.

One consequence of the desire not to be defined by my ailment was that it wasn't necessary to always talk about my health. There were other subjects I was interested in. I have chosen to write this not because I think that is the most important thing for me to be thinking about or the one I most want to talk about, but because my experience may be helpful to others. For some time after I had told the church of my ailment, certain people came up to me with a concerned look and with pitying eyes gazing earnestly into mine said: 'How are you, pastor?' I am grateful for their concern and even more for their prayers but it would have been good to feel that they could think of me other than the 'minister with Parkinson's'. It was a fact of my life I acknowledged openly and shared where I felt was appropriate, but I was not defined by it.

This led me to avoid the usual 'support' groups. As the vast majority of Parkinson sufferers develop the symptoms late in life, most Parkinson's Society groups were made up of folk much older than me and in much more severe stages of the disease. Not wishing to focus my life upon this one aspect or to surround myself with negative images of the effects of the condition, I tried to keep away. I support and am grateful for all those who are committed to helping those of us coping with this ailment and believe the organisations like Parkinson Disease Society do an amazing work which benefit all who are affected by the condition. The same could be said for organisations dedicated to support those with other devastating conditions. The sad truth is that we have become so isolated from each other as a society that finding support in a crisis has to be organised. A good church, however, will enable that support to be given without categorising you or confining you. For example, it gave me **new perspectives** in my situation to sit with others with severe illness, for example, a colleague dying of cancer and someone else needing a spinal operation. This latter was so critical that there was a fifty per cent chance that afterwards he would never walk again. The wider life experiences of others help to give a context to your own that does not diminish it but does prevent you elevating it to a status it does not deserve: this disease is far from the worst thing that could happen to me – bad though it is. It helps, too, with focus. The more important things of life belong elsewhere. Part of handling the responses of others is not to accept the role or image others devise for you. My faith helps in this as I am constantly reminded that my identity is that of a follower of Jesus and child of God. **Ultimately, I will have both a body and a lasting future that does not include Parkinson's or any other disease**.

What then are the songs in the night here? That so many people care. That others who are in need can partner with you in the night and together we can learn to sing. In addition, one of the blessings of having a serious illness is the manner in which you become the focus of many peoples' prayers. A nun, herself far more severely disabled than I have yet experienced, told me she would pray for me five times a day. Others told me they prayed for me every day. This is an amazing privilege and makes at deep and profound levels a great deal of difference. Some expect me to be finally free and totally healed. Their faith may yet carry the day.

If this account so far sounds grim, it is important to relate that it is not the reality we lived in. Good times, even superlatively wonderful times, were still experienced. One of our sons once described us as being a house of laughter. We haven't lost that capacity to see the funny side of things and **the inner joy that is the foundation remains – the underlying melody of songs in the night.**

Chapter 4

SONGS THAT NEED REPEATING
Facing Loss Constantly

'There was evening and there was morning'
(Genesis 1)

The night of tears may pass, but night is followed by day and then the darkness comes down again. Though nothing would be quite as traumatic as that first day in 2001, other days followed when some new loss had to be faced. Progressive disease is particularly subject to this repeated loss, but it is not exclusive to it. The ageing process brings about (differing) degrees of reduced ability; it is greatly multiplied for those with serious and lasting ill-health. Restriction on mobility or on freedom of movement or ease of looking after yourself will mean that a number of opportunities are closed off to the sufferer. Each comes as a new disappointment – an underlining of the limitation imposed on you. In progressive illness, abilities themselves melt away. This attacks the sufferer's self-image. At the same time, our identity is under fire, for we grow used to seeing ourselves in the light of the gifts and abilities we display. To lose one of them is like losing a limb or waking up and finding you have a different face to the one you had only a few days ago – although some might regard this last as a blessing! I wrote of one such loss during a holiday in Scotland. It is a very personal account written just after the events it describes. It does serve to illustrate the point.

My last mountain

Today I said goodbye to the mountain tops, for today I finally admitted defeat. I can no longer tread the high routes to the high peaks and sit on top of the world. My body screams at the effort and I am unsafe on ledges and edges. Slopes make my footing insecure and I am a danger to others as well as myself.

It was not a big mountain, a famous giant. Just Ben Resipol, a Corbett, not a Munro.* To the experienced walker, an easy mountain – for me, Everest. I hadn't felt so bad on the clear, if cloudy, morning. Then my condition, my Parkinson companion, hit. Each movement became an almost unbearable agony that didn't really go away even when stationary. The only relief, if relief it can be called, was when the damaged cells began to choose different parts of the body as the centre of pain. For a while it was my shoulders and neck, and then back to my legs to leaden their mobility.

I wept on Resipol. It first came over me in an uncontrollable wave on a slope that I defied, and in defiance knew that this was my last mountain. I wept for a lost love, a lost ability and a lost delight. I wept because I couldn't do any more what once came so easily and naturally.

Ironically, 'Resipol' means 'homestead'. I had always felt at home in the mountains, those wild and silent places that gave an invigorating, fresh perspective on life. Now their heights were banned. I wept too with Wendy somewhere towards the ridge that led to the summit. Wept at her loss too. I had urged her to go on to the summit without me. She stopped short on the ridge. She had lost her companion of the hills. She too is bereaved and faces a loss.

---

*   A 'Corbett' is a Scottish mountain between 2500ft and 3000ft. A 'Munro' is over 3000ft.

But at least it was magnificent. It was so clear that it seemed that all the Hebridean islands could be seen in one grand sweep. At least the view was good on my last mountain. Ardnamurchan was stretched out below, Loch Sunart and the rest spreading splinters of reflective glass fjord-like through the noble hills. Great peaks jostled and crowded in tiers to the far horizon in the way that seems unique to Scotland. From now on I would gaze up, and not across, to these beautiful places that once I was privileged to be part of. It was how I invariably felt in my heyday – a part of these wondrous heights, drawn into stone and landscape, nature's child hewn together with them by a Creator's hand. I would sit long moments and gaze and be in awe of Him who fashioned and shaped and made such startling and sometimes so fierce a beauty.

The hills are here for a very long haul. My frailty is man's lot – we are outlived by rock and stone. The year before my diagnosis I had climbed to the summits of Ben More Coigach, Ben Dearg, and, most memorably, Suilven. I was exhausted after Coigach but had to turn back on Cul Mor. Determination takes people a long way but it is dangerous to live too much on the edge of your limitations, for these mountains will find you out. The weather can change dramatically. Once climbing Ben Nevis we walked to the top in spectacular sunshine on a crystal clear day. Standing there on the top of Britain and gazing at the huge 360 degree view we saw a cloud carrying a hailstorm approaching. Soon we were glad of every bit of warm and waterproof clothing. To cope with sudden changes in the weather like this or just losing direction there is need to have something in reserve. To always push myself to the limit would be to not only put myself at risk but also others who would be involved in any rescue attempt. Well, maybe I could still walk a little in wild places – on good days. It was thrown into relief by a young couple who parked next to us and preceded us up Ben Resipol. For them it was easy enough – a pleasant day. Enjoy the freedom of the hills whilst it is granted, for all too soon the licence can be revoked.

So, I must learn other pleasures and other worlds – but I will miss the high, silent places where storms rage unchecked and the wind ever blows. Places above the world and its petty strife, a timeless place that works to a long timetable away from human tear and rush. The valley claims me now until another one draws me into its embrace.

So, I somehow worked pedals and wheel and drove us back to our rented croft in the fast-gathering gloom of the evening. We had made it safely down at least, and before dark. Wendy prepared the delights of smoked trout and baby potatoes and corn, and I placed my aching body in bed. The day had drained me of all energy, and the last mountain day closed early.

* * * * * * * * * * *

This is a representative loss of many, some of which are small, some large. Is life, then, just a place of tears? Does the night win out after all? Not at all. There are songs in abundance. As I wrote in the account above, there are other things to discover and other delights to savour. There are, too, compensations.

Somehow the world I experienced had become more sharply focused. It is like the last day at school, rich with vivid moments and fraught with emotions. In fact, I found that my tears flowed more readily and I don't think it was caused by the disease alone. This extra quality added ingredients of depth to experiences and added to the emotions I felt.

The experience of loss also emphasises the fragility of life. The future is never certain and is made more uncertain by the removal of things that are taken for granted. As a result I found myself wanting to take advantage of any opportunity that came my way whilst I could. In some ways, life became fuller because I didn't delay doing things that I really wanted to do until a future date. Even in my work, things that seemed of secondary value rarely gained enough priority to be done. Writing this is part of that.

The story I began to write has a different ending from the one I expected to relate but the urgency came from the impact of the illness. I wanted to write this whilst I knew I could do so and with the hope I might make a contribution to mutual understanding. I wish also to bear witness to the power and amazing kindness of God.

Perhaps our most spectacular opportunity came when unexpectedly we had the chance to go around the world. We had no dreams or plans to make such a trip until some Australian friends, Kerry and Nancy, put the idea into our heads. They were keen for us to visit them in the great land of Oz and one thing led to another and we were even able to spend some time in Hong Kong with one of my brothers. This resulted in us flying from London > Hong Kong > Australia > New Zealand > Fiji > Vancouver > London. This was accomplished in six weeks, during which I managed quite well as far as my health was concerned. I had a few restrictions imposed by the condition with the occasional energy meltdown and the usual aches and pains. I do not remember many days of 'Parkinson slump'. A bonus was that Kerry and Nancy very generously provided us with tickets to the Suncorp Stadium in Brisbane to see England win their quarter final game on the way to winning the Rugby World Cup. The whole trip was bathed in songs of gratitude that we could do such a thing. Had I been fully fit, we may never have done it.

The state of mourning over loss could have become a permanent condition if it had absorbed my attention. Having travelled through the sadness and spilled tears it seemed futile to stay there. The time came to turn from grieving over what I couldn't do, to rejoicing in what I could do. It was not my *disability* but my *ability* or opportunity that had to be where I should concentrate my gaze. This was not always easy because a kind of haze of tiredness descended at times and it was hard to believe it was possible to dredge up energy for anything. I have christened this 'Parkinson slump'. It is common for most Parkinson sufferers, I believe. My own remedy for this, on work days in particular, was to pray and if possible ask someone to pray for me. Then I went out in the faith that in my weakness God would demonstrate His power. Although it may be tempting to avoid people when in this state, being with others seemed to help, not hinder. Despite this, there were days when I seemed to need to rest as much as possible. Should this, however, have been allowed to take control, then I could have sunk into a negative attitude to life. I was determined, however, to stake my faith in God's desire to enable me to live productively and in a way that will be of benefit to others as well as a joy for myself.

In the case of my service for God, my need made me depend all the more on Him and so in some areas I found new ability or effectiveness. It is a Christian basic that God's power is discovered when we depend on Him. The more we rely on Him, the greater our real effectiveness in sharing the grace of God. Physically, to depend on Him to get you through gives a new dimension to this.

Equally, having a major issue of your own can help with a sense of identification with those in need. You have some idea of what it feels like to face these situations. It would be wrong to think, or worse to say, 'I know what you feel like.' The truth is, feelings are individual and everyone's response different. Furthermore, the context is different for each person. By this I mean the background of their life, their present circumstances, their own strength of character, the nature and vibrancy of their faith are factors in how they react. Such things as whether they have a good marriage or not, whether they have learnt to handle pain and hardship in the past are all things that will affect the way they respond. Where my own suffering helped when talking with others with serious illness is in giving a sense of the contours of the landscape of trial. You are able to compare notes, ask some of the right questions, and be aware of some of the little indicators of how people are coping. It is a different way of ministering when you sit **with** someone as a fellow sufferer. It can be legitimate to share some of the things that you find helpful – to comfort others with the comfort you have received, as the apostle Paul would say. It may or may not help, but in sharing we might ourselves discover new help from someone else. There is a companionship in suffering that can be mutually helpful. This is how the best self-help groups work, I think. Anywhere two get together and with honesty share together, there is the potential for encouragement. I believe that this potential is best realised when we have the courage to share more than the facts. We gain most benefit from sharing our feelings, any ways of coping we have adopted and the blessings we have discovered.

In the dark night there comes then the dawn of fresh new light and sometimes these moments are luminous and sharply beautiful. Little things once hardly noticed become treasured. The sight of children playing, the shapes of clouds and the play of light across a landscape can take on a new entrancement. It is as if a little of the stardust of childhood has been sprinkled over the world. Each new loss reawakens this simple joy.

Chapter 5

CHALLENGES TO SONGS IN THE NIGHT

'Why Me?'

In the night, images and questions have room to present themselves, especially when sleep is disturbed by discomfort or pain. What can be silent in the day shouts through the quietness as you try to rest. The questions assert themselves like an unwelcome companion you can't rid yourself of. Loudly insistent, they won't be quiet. The loudest of all was strangely quiet in my company: 'Why me?' I have heard this asked in some form or another by sick people or those near to them over the years and we have wrestled together over the answer. Perhaps this helped equip me to face my own test. Of course there is all the difference in the world between *thinking* of loss and *facing* it. The counsellor does not lose his/her humanity or struggle less with the pain. It is merely that in journeying with others through darkness and doubt I had possibly been given a few signposts to guide me through. I had been, in some measure, prepared then for this particular troublesome guest.

To ask the question 'Why me' is to imply a faith in certain things. Firstly, that there is a god who oversees our lives and therefore what happens in the world. Secondly, such a god is both powerful enough and capable enough to control events in such a way that the outcomes for each individual life are determined. Thirdly, this god also must know everything that is going on. That means a god that is intelligent and personal. To ask 'Why me?' also makes no sense unless you believe this same god wants to make good things happen to you, so this god must be in some measure good. It would be no surprise if your bitterest enemy failed to give you a birthday present. Nor would it amaze you if your father didn't, if you believed he was no longer alive or didn't care for you. You would be disappointed only if you knew he was around and you believed he cared for you. This takes us quite a long way towards the God of the Bible. However, is this all that the Bible says, or does the picture need modifying?

The classic Old Testament book about suffering is Job. In this story a wealthy and godly man who is truly a good man (the story has God Himself give the testimonial) loses everything. In a few short days of extraordinary grief he loses everyone in his household. They are all tragically killed except for his wife and himself. He loses animals, sons and daughters, everyone. Job himself is stricken with a painful and disfiguring illness and his wife tells him to give up, to 'curse God and die.' But Job does not give up. Into this terrifying misery three good friends come and they sit with him. For seven whole days (as mentioned earlier) they say nothing. And then, aided by a clever and younger fourth friend, they seek to help Job. The question they address is: 'Why Job?'

All the statements about God implied by the question, 'Why me?' Job's friends would have endorsed. We would need to add to them their belief that God is perfectly just and fair. As such He metes out in this life His sentence on the way people have conducted themselves. In other words, you get what you deserve in life. This would then mean you could gauge how good a person was by what happened to them in this life. Job's suffering must be because he had done something wrong. 'Admit it, Job, you have looked pretty impressive but the reality is different. Confess.' This argument Job himself rejects. He has done everything he could possibly do to please God. He can't understand why this has happened and wishes there was a way for someone to act as go-between Job and God to plead his case.

This is all carefully worked through in this profound story until God Himself intervenes and speaks. He exonerates Job and reprimands his friends, instructing them to ask Job to pray for them. The clear message is: *Don't judge by either blessing or suffering and trials how God feels about you. God's justice is not completely worked out in this world.*

But God also challenges Job. He does not answer his questions but raises a barrage of His own. 'Were you around when the world was established? How much do you really understand about the world and how it all works?' The questions pile up like a quiz for Nobel Prize winners, except the standard is too high. Job admits defeat and bows humbly before God, awed by the God who answers.

Questions abound around sickness. For example, 'Does Satan or God personally bestow the blessings or trials of life?' Some state, 'This is from Satan,' or 'This is not God's will'. This view seems at first sight to be backed up by the story of Job where Satan actually engineers the suffering. This is not the whole story, though. In Job, Satan only acts by permission of God. God is still in final control. This can be comforting but also serves to reinforce the question: 'So why did He permit this to happen to me?'

Perhaps our perspectives tend to be too individualistic. In the story of Job, his children are all bound up in what is happening to their father. Indeed, the Bible often seems to point to the way in which we are part of family and community. There is a solidarity that means we are affected as a group, not just as individuals. Whole communities are affected by the sins of one man. One example would be Achan in the book of Joshua (Chapter 7). In the midst of battle his covetous greed leads him to take the opportunity to loot a property in the city where the conflict takes place. This action later threatens the whole nation with defeat and disaster.

Classic Christian teaching too accepts this sense of corporate involvement and responsibility. For example, the historic teaching of the church has been that the whole world is affected by the human sinfulness of Adam *'When Adam sinned, sin entered the entire human race. Adam's sin brought death, so death spread to everyone, for everyone sinned.'* (Romans 5:12, NLT.) The only remedy for this is to be involved in what Jesus has done and be part of His new community. *'The sin of this one man, Adam, caused death to rule over us, but all who receive God's wonderful, gracious gift of righteousness will live in triumph over sin and death through this one man, Jesus Christ.'* (Romans 5:17, NLT.)* Or, on another occasion, *'Everyone dies because all of us are related to Adam, the first man. But all who are related to Christ, the other man, will be given new life.'* (1 Corinthians 15:22, NLT.) In the same way, we are caught up today in the injustice, war and violence of others. Many people, for example, who were opposed to the 2003 war on Iraq were nevertheless touched by it. Similarly, many opposed to Saddam Hussein in Iraq suffered because of his sins. Some were tragically affected by the human rights violations that brought them so much suffering, others from the economic impact of their international isolation, and still others as innocent victims of the Gulf wars. Terrorists, by design, involve innocent bystanders in their violent conflicts and hatreds. For the USA, their first experience of this was the destruction of the World Trade Centre on '9/11' (11 September 2001). The rest of the world sympathetically welcomed them into suffering humanity and the reality that the innocent suffer. We are not taken out of this arena of human follies before death and inevitably have to share the pains, with others, of our human tragedies. We are bound up together in life. Sickness and

---

*   *Holy Bible: New Living Translation*. 1997. Wheaton, Ill.: Tyndale House.

ill-health are no different. Jesus identified with a broken and sinful world. It should be no surprise that we find ourselves a part of it too. I become sick because I am woven into the fabric of this damaged world.

As ever, Jesus casts a clear light on our questions. In John chapter 9 we are told of a man born blind. Catching sight of him begging beside the road, the disciples ask, 'Who sinned, this man or his parents?' What is the point of such a question? Simply because they carried the same assumptions that were expressed by Job's friends; namely that sickness is caused by personal sin. The man was blind, they thought, because God was measuring out a just punishment. But as he was **born** blind, whose sin was it? Did he sin in the womb, or was it judgement on his parents that their son should be afflicted? Jesus replied: 'Neither this man nor his parents sinned.' He quashes the idea that all sickness is caused by sin. Some may be, but not all. Jesus added, 'so that the work of God may be displayed in His life.'

It is this attitude that I felt was key to my own sickness. Somehow God will gain glory in it. My personal response was therefore to yield my life up to God for Him to glorify His name whether as a Parkinson sufferer or not. I have no rights in this – it is He Who determines what happens in the future and it will be good. Which brings us back to Job.

The story begins with a dramatic encounter between God and the Devil. God points to the wonderful character of Job. The Devil counters with the accusation that the only reason Job was faithful to God was because God gave him so many good things, 'but take them away and then he would soon curse you.' Job had every reason to trust God, Satan argued; it was 'good for business'. He added, 'Let Job lose these material benefits then see just how faithless he is'. God accepted the challenge and allowed the Devil to bring tragedy into Job's life. But Job still loved God even when everything was taken away. So another confrontation took place between Satan and God. 'Let me touch his own body *and he will curse You soon enough,*' claims Satan. Again he is given his wish. But though Job questions, he remains faithful.

This raises a challenging issue. Is our faith only 'feel-good' deep? Are we believers just for the blessing? If, like Jesus, we had to face some sort of cross, would we turn and run, or go through with it as He did? If I am sick and remain unhealed, shall I curse my Saviour and reject Him? Or do I have the kind of faith that remains faithful in trial?

The story of Job makes him totally unaware of the challenge which takes place in the court of heaven. This, I suggest, indicates the truth that there are things going on we cannot possibly know or totally understand. We need to accept our ignorance. Let us trust God, knowing He will not let us down even if we do not understand right now.

The book finishes with a final triumph and restoration for Job. Some take the view that this is an inappropriate ending and has been tacked on. I, however, found such hope an essential part of my armoury in trouble. It speaks of a God who is good and therefore will bless, however grim the immediate present is. That blessing may begin here in this life but will ultimately be ours in heaven, in eternal glory. Whatever we go through here, it is worth bearing if we reach there. 'Yet *what we suffer now is nothing compared to the glory he will give us later.*' (Romans 8:18, NLT.)

The answer to the original question 'Why me?' is then 'To glorify God'. In that spirit, it offers opportunity for a special sacrifice of devoted praise. We can take this circumstance to serve God, not for what we get out of Him, but simply because we love Him. We place ourselves in position to do that as we trust in a God Who is always faithful to us.

Philippians 1:20-21 (NLT)

For I live in eager expectation and hope that I will never do anything that causes me shame, but that I will *always be bold for Christ, as I have been in the past, and that my life will always honor Christ, whether I live or I die. For to me, living is for Christ, and dying is even better.**

---

* *Holy Bible: New Living Translation.* 1997. Wheaton, Ill.: Tyndale House.

Chapter 6

THE SONG THAT BANISHED THE NIGHT

Some Release from Sickness

I began to feel I had been healed on 22 April 2004. It happened at a 'routine' breakfast-time prayer meeting of Southwark ministers in London when Pastor Sam Larbie gave testimony of the way God had been healing people and sought to share how to encourage others in this ministry. His slogan is 'Healing is easy because of what Jesus has done' and is the title of a short book he has written.

To put this into context, the year had started badly for me. The days of 'Parkinson slump', a kind of depression, had increased and the exhaustion had grown. I had constant muscle pain and stiffness and fought through tiredness. This last problem was not helped by my failure to sleep more than three or four hours at a time. I would wake up with legs, shoulders, and right arm in particular aching and stiff. By mid-April I usually woke up with two or three fingers in my right hand being rigid and immovable. I had to massage them to get them to function at all. Sometimes this was Wendy's first duty of the day and occasionally she would massage my aching legs too. I had begun to ask, 'Lord, do You want me to continue in this ministry? Show me what to do next.' I couldn't properly see what that future might be.

On that morning in April, Sam said, 'I don't want to be a star but to teach my people how to pray for the sick and be involved in the healing ministry.'

So he demonstrated. 'Let's hold hands – and pray after me.' He was holding my right hand. 'This belongs to me because of what Jesus has done. I receive my healing now in Jesus' name,' he said. I wondered a little about the theology, but joined in as we all prayed, using Sam's words.

After the prayer, I didn't notice much that was different but listened as Sam went on to explain the prayer. He told us he received these words after praying for guidance over how he could encourage his people to pray for the sick. He teaches this particular prayer to everyone who will listen. 'So, let's pray it again.' We did. He told us some more stories of people being healed in the street and in shops here in London. He presented a fascinating and sometimes amusing picture of his shopping expeditions to Tesco's:

'I will meet someone and ask, "Do you know Jesus loves you?" Then I ask, "Do you have a pain somewhere?" When they say, "Yes," I ask them to pray after me...'

He then repeated the prayer and got us to do the same once more. Apparently he had seen a stream of people healed in this way. 'Once I used to sweat and work so hard for people to be healed. But this is so easy,' he said. I chipped in that you don't have to shout for God to hear you. These were simple, quietly spoken prayers.

Earlier, someone in the meeting suggested that the group should pray for me, but the only specific prayer was offered amongst many other issues relating to Southwark. I went away feeling somewhat disappointed that there had been no real follow-up on the proposal, but I was also moved by the apparent effectiveness of Sam's healing ministry and wanted to work out what we could learn from it. What I did notice as I walked down the road was how free my right hand was. In fact, I realised I was feeling well all through my body. I continued like that all day. Could God have healed me after all? But how would

I know this? Furthermore, if I was healed, could I safely come off the medication? I had little or no time to follow up these concerns as some difficult pastoral issues were raised immediately after the meeting which dominated the day and left me somewhat disturbed. There was no surrounding circumstance to suggest some psychological explanation for what happened next.

When at last I had time to think and pray about how I was feeling, I realised that there was little actual experience out there of the situation I was in. Parkinson's disease is medically speaking incurable and there are no remissions, only deterioration, at different rates, but ever on a downward slope. As a result, rightly or wrongly, I decided that medical advice would not help me much. In consultation with Wendy, a trained nurse, I decided on a course of action. To begin with, I would do nothing but monitor my health over a few days so that I could be sure I wasn't just enjoying a good day after so many bad ones. In myself I had confidence that in fact my sense of well-being was more than this. If all was still well I would then slowly try to take myself off the medication. The reasoning behind this was that the body needed to adjust to producing all its own dopamine again. Dopamine is normally produced by the body, but in Parkinson sufferers this is increasingly reduced. This is the real cause of the slow paralysis that creeps over the body. The drug levodopa is given to provide a substitute and reduce the symptoms. I therefore came to the conclusion that I should only ease off the drugs slowly.

Over the next few days my sense of physical well-being continued and improved. On 26 April, I reduced the night-time medication for the first time. That day we had gone out for a walk and accidentally forgot to take any tablets with us. We were delighted to do an undulating six miles with me having no difficulties at all. Afterwards I drove home without problems of tiredness or aches and pains. I arrived at home at 4:30 pm still feeling well where, the week before, I would have been totally exhausted. Even the following day I had no ill effects. I had not felt like this for years but did not want to 'go public' until I could demonstrate that this was not just a feeling or a state of mind. I needed to be able to testify clearly and powerfully so that there was no reasonable doubt about what God had done.

The significance of that walk is highlighted when we compare this experience with earlier in the year when I had attempted a country walk on a quiet road. The road had been fairly flat with few undulations and the whole distance about four miles. As usual, my body went through various degrees of discomfort and pain and a migraine began to develop. These had afflicted me with increasing frequency during the year. They were not particularly painful but affected my sight so much that I could only lie down quietly and wait for them to pass. Any activity just made them worse. So it was a relieved man who very wearily reached the little café at the end of the walk and sat down to recover. Before 22 April, even gentle country walks like this were under threat. Yet four days after the prayer meeting, I took this more arduous walk in my stride and finished bounding in energy. A true transformation had taken place.

The day after that walk, I stopped taking cabergolin altogether. I had been taking this for about three years and my consultant had been easing me off it already because of side effects. It has a different medical purpose from levodopa and is intended to delay the use of levo-dopa or enhance its effectiveness. I was still taking levo-dopa, which was the main drug used in my treatment at that stage.

At this point I again turn to records I wrote at the time.

Thurs 29 April 04. Today I awake to celebrate my first week clear of aches and pains for years. Yesterday I had worked hard moving office furniture as we re-organised the church offices, had an evening meeting and walked to pray and minister to someone in hospital who had been dying of cancer. Her family were also present. Since we had been praying for her she had been making a remarkable recovery. I had not stopped all day, and had talked to her family, who were staying with us, until midnight. This is recorded to indicate just how well I am. I am up and about the next day with no adverse effects and my body feels loose and free and normal. During the last week I have at no time felt the kind of muscle pain that I have lived with every day for the last few years. I no longer had stiffness when sitting in one position or the exhausted 'wasted' feeling in my muscles when walking. I cannot say I have never felt any stiffness, but what little I have had has quickly passed. I realise just how much I have had to fight against tiredness and that depressing cloud that settled over me. Not for a minute this whole week have I felt that, but have been fully alive and alert. It is an awesome and wonderful experience to have my body begin to work normally again. I was amazed to discover that I had to relearn how to do things. For example I had become used to using my left hand and now I can go back to using my right. This is the most amazing thing. My right hand had been so clumsy and my fingers seemed fat and unresponsive but now feel slim and more agile. I don't think I have full return to complete ability yet but they are astonishingly different. Tomorrow I shall reduce my levodopa for the first time. I believe the Lord told me that I will not be totally healed until all the drugs are finished with. I just want to worship Him. I had begun to have doubts about even driving up to Scotland for our holiday but now I have no anxieties about that and I am thinking about mountains again.

30 April 2004 I had my morning dose of levodopa only, having forgotten about the evening one. I have had no ill effects of this. As a consequence I will keep it that way for a week before dropping them altogether.

3 May 2004 I am still doing well and clear of symptoms. My energy levels are up and I seem to feel better at the end of the drug time. (That is, the further from the time of taking tablets, the better I seem.) I have just had a full 7-8 hours of sleep and have woken up comfortably in bed. I have not done that for years it seems. When I was ill if I had a better night's sleep, I used to wake up very stiff the next day. I had resorted to taking a dose of levodopa and cabergolin as late at night as possible to enable me to sleep longer. I don't recall ever sleeping more than 5 hours at a stretch whatever I did. This was happening in the weeks leading up to the healing.

5 May 2004 I took my very last Parkinson tablets today.

The following weeks were a wonderful joy to me as I exulted in living drug free and without pain. On my days off I was enjoying walking again unhindered by Parkinson stiffness and other symptoms. From this time onwards, my energy and physical capabilities were transformed. Even though I was taking no medication of any kind I was sleeping better – even up to eight hours. More importantly, I never once woke up aching or stiff at all. Since 22 April all morning massage was totally unnecessary. I woke up totally free of pains and aches. My muscles were loose and I was comfortable just lying in bed. I could even sleep on my side, which I could not do at all before as I would soon get very stiff and it would be too painful or uncomfortable. Furthermore, I had had to sleep on a mound of pillows to aid my breathing. I soon found myself far more comfortable on one or two pillows at most. On one walk I experienced an unexpected pleasure – I smelt the wild flowers. That was the first realisation that my sense of smell had returned to me. My food too began to have more taste.

On 17 May I had what may have seemed a setback – another migraine. I had at least one each week before 22 April, and they struck unpredictably. Just before my healing I had had three in 24 hours. I could be walking down the road or just sitting in my chair and suddenly I began to feel odd and a strange weaving 'filament' of bright light would impede the sight over half my field of vision. This latest migraine was only the second since 22 April.

My physical condition changed so much that when on 29 May we attended a family wedding; we planned a weekend of walks whilst we stayed on a Northampton-shire farm. On the Sunday (30 May) I walked five rough country miles before breakfast and 10 miles in total that day, very comfortably. The Monday was a glorious day. Wendy and I had a wonderful walk on the ridge tops near the lovely Leicestershire village of Hallaton. That beautiful day we walked 13 miles and ran the last part! This was out of elation and fun since our Father had given back to us a precious gift we thought had been taken away for ever. I had no aches and pains and no difficulties. We were able to enjoy a canal-side stroll the next morning before heading back to London. I didn't even have the normal muscle stiffness I might have expected from such sudden return to exercise. This is typical of the days that followed.

It was not until 6 June 2004 that I told the church of my healing. In the previous weeks, a number had been telling me how well I looked. When I explained what had happened, they could see it plainly enough in my whole posture, freedom of movement, voice and facial expres-sion and appearance. The testimony was clearly to be seen as well as heard. The response was dynamic.

Earlier I have written about loss and how in progressive disease the sufferer faces not one loss but repeated loss. Now, with so much of my energy and ability restored, I had the delight of renewing acquaintance with joys that had seemed to be denied to me for ever. One such was walking amongst my beloved mountains. We drove to Scotland and took the ferry to the Outer Hebrides (or Western Isles as they are called today). There I recorded the following:

23 June 2004 Return to the mountains.

Today I did the impossible. On this day I returned to the mountains, or the mountains were returned to me. On Resipol in 2002 I wept at the loss of another part of my life as I said goodbye to the mountains, unable to climb any more. On this morning I wept to think I could seriously contemplate climbing Clisham.

I had had this in mind ever since I had been healed. We had already arranged our Hebridean trip and Clisham is the highest mountain in the Western Isles. At 2621 ft or 799m it may not rank as a Munro, but at our age, and coming after a lengthy illness, testing enough. The ground, in this very wet year, was energy-sapping bog. The higher slopes are steep and the final stretch along a ridge. There were moments when I wondered if we would make it. High up I prayed 'Should I go on?' The reply seemed to be a firm 'Yes – step by step as in everything. You will reach the goal even as you will in the greater challenge in London.' So we climbed up and along the ridge in cloud, found the trig point surrounded by its wall and were quietly exultant. The way down was taxing and we fell and slipped more than once in the heather, from tiredness mostly. But we could laugh for there were no Parkinson pains or stiffness, just normal healthy weariness. I recovered well and felt only a normal stiffness. In fact I am beginning to wonder when I did last feel so well. So, this gift was given us – the mountains have been returned to us both. What an amazing God we worship!

I drove over 1900 miles over two weeks of holiday and we walked when we could. It was hard to remember when I last felt so well.

So how complete is my healing? I feel that nearly everything I have lost over recent years has been restored to me. I am astonished now to realise just how many body functions were affected by my illness. However, it has left me with some residual reminders of my former trials which surface most clearly when I am tired. These focus mostly on my right hand which is still not as able and nimble as it was. At no point since 22 April have I had a return of the cramps, aches and pains, and 'slump' days I suffered before. In fact, I am now compared favourably by some with others of my age group who have no illness or disability. I am told I have an energy and level of activity that others might envy. This is not to boast – I can point to plenty of others of my age that leave me standing. It is merely an indication of how much vigour and energy has been restored. This restored ability largely continued until I retired in 2012.

People have asked me how members of the medical profession have responded to all this. The Christian ones who know me have been both delighted and encouraged by my story. There were a number of health professionals in my congregation, including eminent ones, who rejoiced with everyone else at what was clear to see before their eyes. My own consultant at King's College Neurological Department saw me on the 21 July. He affirmed that I was doing all the right things in the circumstances. He said he thought I should stay off medication 'unless I really wanted to take something.' I was happy to stay drug-free. He also said that he detected some residual signs of Parkinson's disease and wished to see me in six-seven months. (These residual signs I have already mentioned.) I left him with much to think about. It is worth noting that no cases of spontaneous remission in Parkinson sufferers exist nor could anyone give any medical reason for my improvement. If any treatment or drug therapy had the same results, it would bring worldwide acclaim and make headline news. The most that doctors treating Parkinson's disease hope for is to slow down the inexorable march of this terrible disorder. The search for a cure continues, as does the search for the cause. I pray they will both succeed, but nobody heals as well as Jesus my Lord.

I have been asked if I believe I have been healed for ever. I hope and pray the symptoms never return but I can only testify to how I am now. The future is not mine to command but I am confident that God will not fail me. He has not failed me in all the years I have served Him and I have no reason to doubt Him now. I was 15 years old when I fully committed my life to Christ and I am awed by what

God has done for me today. I know how different I feel now from the years prior to 22 April 2004. Tomorrow is in His hands.

Postscript

As I review this in 2020, I can say that I have deteriorated gradually during retirement. I have lived longer than my father or my grandfather, despite my condition. To date I have lived 19 years with the threat of Parkinson's since diagnosis. In spite of a return to slow deterioration, I believe God has a purpose for me and His joy remains. I can only respond by echoing Mary's song of joy.

My, how God has blessed me
Based on Luke 1:46-55

'I just can't stop telling you how wonderful the Lord is.
I am bursting with joy because of God my Saviour.
For he even took notice of me, his undistinguished servant,
and now people can see how He has blessed me.
For He, the Mighty One, is holy, and He has done great things
   for me.
His mercy and kindness continues through the generations, to
   all who trust and revere Him.
In His might He does tremendous things! He has forgiven my
   sins and healed my sickness. He has restored me body and
   soul.
How He humiliates the proud and arrogant!
How He dethrones the powerful of this world
and honours the people no one thought about.
He has satisfied the hungry with good things
and sent the rich away with empty hands.
And how He has helped his servant people!
He has not forgotten His promise to be merciful.*

For He promised to send His Spirit just as He did to the
  apostles and prophets –
to display His mercy to them and through them forever.'
How good is our God and how precious Jesus our Saviour. How
  marvellous the gift of His Spirit.
Surely we could just praise Him all day long and even night
  time wouldn't dampen our spirits.
Come and praise the Lord with me and glorify Him all day
  every day.

Chapter 7

SONGS OF HOPE IN THE NIGHT

Jesus And Healing Today

Perhaps one of the most striking experiences of healing I have come across took place amongst a Church in Siberia. The church had arranged for myself and a colleague to teach their leaders. The city where we ministered was an industrial, polluted city not very far from Mongolia. It was an independent, evangelical church, which had grown very quickly in its eight years of existence. It had birthed a number of daughter churches in the area surrounding this steel town. Inside the city itself, the church was about 1,000-strong. The leadership team was also substantial, and it was to these leaders we were tasked to bring some greater grasp of Christian teaching and further application of their faith. This they eagerly took to, using any scrap of paper they could find to take notes. There was an awareness on our part that they would seek to act on what was being taught.

Each day followed a particular pattern. After we had gone through a block of teaching, we were almost always asked to pray for some who were sick. They had little access to quality medical help – 'We only have Jesus,' they said. Later, I sought to enquire what had happened as a result of our prayers. They looked at me rather strangely as if I had asked a ridiculous question. They had been healed, of course: what else? There was no drama, just a quiet expectation that God would meet them in their need. In reflecting on this, I was very aware of how different their situation and ours is. Spiritually they live in a dynamic and powerful time of growth and encounter with God by the Holy Spirit. They are a people who have a wholehearted and passionate commitment to Christ. Far from perfect, nevertheless their need makes them aware of their dependence on God in a way foreign to our experience in the West. Physically, their society lives on the edge of destruction. If the communal heating plants and infrastructure do not work in their fierce winter months, then these tough Siberian people will die. Yet everything is creaking with age and totters close to breakdown. Not far away is the vast forest wilderness that is the backdrop of many of their lives. (The church pastor hunted bears!) It lends a stern background note of the battle to survive, a primitive struggle for existence. In such a context, faith rises and abandonment to God is easier to come by. I would suggest that God is moved by such extremity and meets such folk in a special way in their need and their faith.

Interestingly, at the time I visited Siberia it is likely that I had been suffering Parkinson's disease for some three years but that it had not yet been diagnosed. I was not particularly aware of the symptoms at that time but I am grateful that I was able to minister healing even though ill myself. The probability is that I developed the illness soon after I moved to London early in 1998.

I am aware that, for many people, stories of divine healing in distant Eastern Siberia are less than convincing. So what took place on my return and how about healings nearer to home? Here, too, I have met people who tell of their own experience of healing. One lady told me that she had been through the terrible trauma of going blind. Some time later she was at a worship service, the focus of which was to praise and glorify God. Deeply moved, and not asking God for anything, she slowly began to realise that she could see again. She took great delight in pointing out the pillar where she had stood for support and said: 'As I *was praising God, slowly my sight returned.*'

Another healing about eyesight in which I was more directly involved concerned a fellow minister. A group of us met monthly to pray and talk of our ministry or whatever was relevant to us. One newish member told us that he had just been told that the back of his eye was in such a poor state that he would lose his sight altogether in that eye in the following few days. We prayed specifically that his sight should be saved and his eye healed. He had been given an urgent return appointment, where it was discovered that the deterioration had been reversed and his sight saved. I know some will treat these accounts with some scepticism, or look for some naturalistic explanation. For my part I can only record honestly what I have seen and heard. Nevertheless you might justifiably ask: 'What about you and your Parkinson's?' In response I return to my account of my own life experience.

Our return trip home from Siberia was an adventure in itself. The first sign that anything out of the ordinary had occurred was when it was announced on our Air France flight from Moscow to Paris that they didn't have any wine! They had been delayed by storms and they just didn't have the time to load all the supplies. This surprising admission amazed us since the stereotypical Frenchman would have loaded the wine first! Some very large Russians drank their own vodka instead. This we found somewhat troubling. Despite this concern, we were safely delivered as far as France. When we landed at Charles de Gaulle airport in Paris it was in chaos. We found it almost impossible to get any reliable information of our flight home. Eventually we managed to board a flight to the UK and very late in the day made it back to our respective homes.

The return trip, for me, was a trial of endurance, as I had developed a fluey cold. This persisted for longer than I expected, so a visit to the doctor seemed a sensible course of action. At the end of the consultation, I said somewhat apologetically that I also had a stiff arm. It was not very painful but was uncomfortable. After examination, the GP arranged an appointment for me with a neurology specialist at King's College hospital.

This apparently world-renowned specialist was compassionate and careful. Having run a series of tests, he delivered the verdict, which is where this book started. As many a Christian has discovered, God frequently acts as an alchemist of the soul, turning the dark places, and painful places, into places of undiscovered blessing. In my case, what I came to think of as 'Siberian flu' brought about the diagnosis which may not otherwise have happened. I would probably have struggled on undiagnosed and increasingly incapable of fulfilling my ministry. Yet a question was left hanging in the air: 'How long would I be able to continue in this work?' I believe that the chain of events that led to my diagnosis, and by world-renowned specialists at that, was the result of God's intervention. '*He [God] gives yet more grace*' (NIV) and gives the strength to tread the path ahead with hope and no little joy.

I hope that the testimonies I have related leave the open-minded observer in little doubt that in Jesus' name people are healed today in Britain. **In case anyone doubts the original diagnosis,** I would point out that, as I have already noted, it was made by top specialists at King's College Hospital, London. Furthermore, through a set of circumstances, the initial diagnosis was confirmed by another top specialist. He took great care to check that I had Parkinson's disease and not something else that gave similar symptoms. I make this point again to clarify the medical situation. Personally I can only tell you the effects of a simple and quiet prayer that made an immediate and complete change to my physical well-being. For three years I lived with a diagnosed condition that was progressively taking a hold of me and affecting every part of my body. I joked once that soon I would make the acquaintance of every medical department in those hospitals that treated me for the various problems that arose. (I was also treated at Guy's and St Thomas'.) The medical person who

received this comment said encouragingly: 'You probably will over the next few years.' Such was the nature of
my condition that at no time day or night was I free from
aches, pains and some impairment of my ability to do
things. This changed from the moment I was prayed for
in that room on 22 April 2004. Since then the aches and
pains have disappeared and the different disabilities were
either gradually or immediately restored to normal ability.
In other words, I know the difference every moment of
every day and I am awed to be the subject of such amazing
grace.

I think it important to say that I would not normally
advocate anyone coming off medication 'in faith' without
medical advice. I have already indicated why and how I did
so myself. It also needs to be mentioned that when I was
ill to miss tablets would have real physical consequences
quite quickly. I would soon have known about it if nothing
had changed. Furthermore, I would have severe discomfort – but my life would not be not in danger. I would have
taken a different course of action under different circumstances and if I had been suffering another kind of illness. I
regard the medical profession as allies in the battle against
sickness. I also felt well for some time before taking any
action. Faith is not about pretence. I believed God would
give me a healing that was clear enough for me to take
sensible decisions. We don't need to presume or assume
things to demonstrate our faith. For three years I took the
medication as prescribed.

My particular healing though raises **the issue of divine
healing in general.** Is it for all who will receive it by faith?
I personally believe that God's intention is to bring health
and wholeness to us all through the work of Jesus. This
means far more than good physical health – it also means
spiritual health and eternal life and a whole lot more. All
these things hang together. For example, to be healed of
a stress-related illness, as high blood pressure can be, is
a blessing. Wouldn't it be far better if it is also combined
with the trust in God that deals with the stress as well? Or

to be healed of a sexually transmitted disease is wonderful. However, doesn't any immoral lifestyle need to be forgiven and the lifestyle changed to a God pleasing moral one? The very word 'health' comes from an Old English root *hail* which means 'whole, entire, unimpaired'. The words 'wholeness' and 'holiness' are both derived from this same Old English base. The World Health Organisation defined health as 'a state of complete physical, mental and social well-being and not merely the absence of disease and infirmity.' Jesus speaks of bringing fullness of life, '*My purpose is to give life in all its fullness*' (John 10:10, NLT).* This life is one made and sustained only in relationship to God through Jesus His Son. '*And this is the way to have eternal life—to know you, the only true God, and Jesus Christ, the one you sent to earth*' (John 17:3, NLT).† So to be truly healthy is to be well in body, mind and spirit with wholesome relationships both human and divine.‡ In the New Testament the word meaning 'to save' is used of both physical and spiritual healing.

It is for good reason then that when the apostle James talks of healing prayer he includes confession of sins:

'*Are any among you sick? They should call for the elders of the church and have them pray over them, anointing them with oil in the name of the Lord. And their prayer offered in faith will heal the sick, and the Lord will make them well. And anyone who has committed sins will be forgiven. Confess your sins to each other and pray for each other so that you may be healed. The earnest prayer of a righteous person has great power and wonderful results*' (James 5:14-16, NLT).§

---

* Holy Bible: New Living Translation. 1997. Wheaton, Ill.: Tyndale House.

† Holy Bible: New Living Translation. 1997. Wheaton, Ill.: Tyndale House.

‡ See article on 'Healing' New Dictionary of Theology (2000) Ferguson, S. B., & Packer, J. InterVarsity Press,

§ Holy Bible: New Living Translation. 1997. Wheaton, Ill.: Tyndale House.

One component of physical sickness may or may not be spiritual, but nobody is truly whole who remains estranged from God. Confession of sin and real repentance are part of entering or restoring that relationship, which means changes in our life. A great many of the illnesses we suffer in the West are caused by lifestyle and our inner attitudes. If we let Christ transform these, then perhaps we would live healthier lives. Maybe a different kind of healing is required then for many in the West. But aren't changes in lifestyle and attitude the very things we resist the most?

If good health is more than freedom from disease and infirmity, then 'spiritual healers' who do not heal in the name of Jesus and do not encourage confession of our failure to live as God would have us live cannot bring the wholeness that only Jesus can provide, whatever their claims. Such necessary confession, if combined with a real confidence in God's forgiving love, can lead to a more wholesome way of living. Added to this is the inner peace that remains in all that we go through. It is not surprising that some have found themselves brought into a new set of spiritual problems by resorting to such 'healers' in desperation. Why are we so slow or reluctant to bring our desperation to our loving heavenly Father? Similarly, just turning to medical practitioners without also seeking Christian counsel and prayer is surely also to miss an essential part of God's healing purpose for us. We are more than biological 'machines' that go wrong from time to time and need good biomechanics to sort it all out. To meet our real need, all our sickness should be treated.

A kind of theological slogan states that 'healing is in the atonement'. Although sometimes misused or even potentially misleading, I believe this phrase is essentially correct. The statement expresses the truth that in dying for us Jesus brings 'good health' or the wholeness of body, mind and spirit outlined above. The ultimate purpose of God is to remove the curse of sin, sickness and separation from God. This is expressed graphically in the last book of the Bible, Revelation:

> 'Then I saw a new heaven and a new earth, for the old heaven and the old earth had disappeared. And the sea was also gone. And I saw the holy city, the new Jerusalem, coming down from God out of heaven like a beautiful bride prepared for her husband. I heard a loud shout from the throne, saying, "Look, the home of God is now among his people! He will live with them, and they will be his people. God himself will be with them. He will remove all of their sorrows, and there will be no more death or sorrow or crying or pain. For the old world and its evils are gone forever."' (Revelation 21:1-4, NLT.)

> 'And the angel showed me a pure river with the water of life, clear as crystal, flowing from the throne of God and of the Lamb, coursing down the center of the main street. On each side of the river grew a tree of life, bearing twelve crops of fruit, with a fresh crop each month. The leaves were used for medicine to heal the nations. No longer will anything be cursed. For the throne of God and of the Lamb will be there, and his servants will worship him.' (Revelation 22:1-3, NLT.)*

I believe this blessing can only be ours because Jesus willingly died for us on the cross. In dying and rising again, Jesus overcame the powers of evil, including sin and death – together with their ally, sickness. I can only be part of this through truly trusting Him in His kindness to give me this wonderful gift. It is never something I can say I deserve.

This, then, is God's future for His people. But not all of this is present now. When Jesus came He had an agenda

---

* *Holy Bible: New Living Translation.* 1997. Wheaton, Ill.: Tyndale House.

that included healing the sick – the beginning of this new era where heaven invades earth:

> 'The Spirit of the Lord is upon me, for he has appointed me to preach Good News to the poor. He has sent me to proclaim that captives will be released, that the blind will see, that the downtrodden will be freed from their oppressors, and that the time of the Lord's favour has come.' (Luke 4:18-19, NLT.)*

When Jesus healed and delivered people, we see His Kingdom entering our world. In fact, every time some evil is overcome in Jesus' name and some life is saved or restored it is an extending of God's Kingdom. So Jesus sends the disciples out with this commission – 'Go and announce to them that the Kingdom of Heaven is near. Heal the sick, raise the dead, cure those with leprosy, and cast out demons. Give as freely as you have received!' (Matthew 10:7-8, NLT.) † That the apostles saw healing as part of their Christian mission after Pentecost is shown by their practice. They did include these things in their ministry and so should we. I believe that to fail to do so is to fall short of the commission Christ has given us. Throughout its history, the church has recognised this as an element in its ministry. For example, from the fourth century onwards Christians have run hospitals. This is in itself not very controversial.

More controversial is the claim that Christians can and do bring physical healing through prayer alone. This too has a long history. Apart from the events of the New Testament we have references like this one from Cyril of Jerusalem (348–386 AD), a respected bishop:

---

* *Holy Bible: New Living Translation.* 1997. Wheaton, Ill.: Tyndale House.

† *Holy Bible: New Living Translation.* 1997. Wheaton, Ill.: Tyndale House.

'Jesus then means according to the Hebrew "Saviour," but in the Greek tongue "The Healer"; since He is physician of souls and bodies, curer of spirits, curing the blind in body, and leading minds into light, healing the visibly lame, and guiding sinners' steps to repentance, saying to the palsied, Sin no more, and, Take up thy bed and walk. For since the body was palsied for the sin of the soul, He ministered first to the soul that He might extend the healing to the body. If, therefore, any one is suffering in soul from sins, there is the Physician for him: and if anyone here is of little faith, let him say to Him, Help Thou mine unbelief. If any is encompassed also with bodily ailments, let him not be faithless, but let him draw nigh; for to such diseases also Jesus ministers, and let him learn that Jesus is the Christ.'*

Similar statements or allusions are made in Christian writings in the early centuries of the church. Later records also make claim to healings; for example, Donald Bridges notes that Bede's *The Ecclesiastical History of the English People* is 'shot full of the miraculous.'† Bede is described as a quiet, pious and scholarly man living in north-east England in the 7th and 8th centuries. Such testimony is sometimes belittled or ignored – but still remains as witness to the awareness that healing prayer is part of the Christian mission. It is in more 'modern' centuries that this call has been muted.

If we see little happen as a result of our prayers we need to ask why. Is there something that needs correcting, perhaps? Has God taken authority away from us so that we might feel impelled to seek Him urgently and humbly? Perhaps James 4 has an important message for us:

---

*   Schaff, P. (1997). *The Nicene and Post-Nicene Fathers Second Series Vol. VII. Cyril of Jerusalem, Gregory Nazianzen*. Oak Harbor: Logos Research Systems.

†   Donald Bridge *'Signs and wonders today'* p161. 1985 IVP

'And even when you do ask, you don't get it because your whole motive is wrong—you want only what will give you pleasure.' (James 4:3.) 'Draw close to God, and God will draw close to you. Wash your hands, you sinners; purify your hearts, you hypocrites. Let there be tears for the wrong things you have done. Let there be sorrow and deep grief. Let there be sadness instead of laughter, and gloom instead of joy.' (James 4:8-9, NLT.)

For some years now, Christian leaders from Britain have visited countries overseas and found themselves ministering with a new freedom and power. Returning home, they attempt the same things but haven't seen the same results. Healings can be rare, non-existent or infrequent. I feel the churches of the West have grown used to seeing only small signs of God's miraculous power and regard it as normal Christianity. The tendency is to treat reports from other parts of the world that speak of miracles and healings as dubious, or maybe even the sad delusions of a primitive people. So when the stories come to us from some materially poor country that read like pages from the New Testament book of Acts, we believe them to be exaggerated, superstitious or just lying. Instead of questioning ourselves, we question the gospel and re-interpret the promises and commands of God so that they mean something other than what has been plainly written. We have been guilty of theologically taming the gospel and robbing it of its power. We have rationalised the dynamic God of the Bible into a pale and feeble image of our own. If I have come out of this experience with anything, it is the deep conviction that it is time for us to take the awesome God of the Bible seriously.

As I sit in wonder at the God Who restored me, I am fully aware that I was made well only because of what Jesus has done and not because of any quality in me. What made it possible was His terrible suffering on the cross. This is the reason we can have hope. He died voluntarily to bear the suffering I deserve and to carry the consequences of my sin. He willingly gives us what we don't deserve. By the same power that Jesus was raised to life out of that death, we can be freed from sin and its consequences. The same goes for healing. In other words we can be healed in spite of our sin. We can, in fact, have a whole fresh start with a new strength to enable us to succeed where we once failed so badly.

This does not mean that I believe every person prayed for will be immediately healed. For over three years I was prayed for and was not healed. I was sustained but slowly deteriorated. The authority to bring healing will not mean everybody will be made well here in this life. I notice that Jesus also sent the apostles to raise the dead, some were, but the cemeteries were not emptied. In the same way not all will be healed though many will be. In Jesus' ministry there were special times when healing power seemed to be present: '*Everyone was trying to touch him, because healing power went out from him, and they were all cured.*' (Luke 6:19, NLT.) At others less took place, for example at Nazareth: '*And because of their unbelief, he couldn't do any mighty miracles among them except to place his hands on a few sick people and heal them.*' (Mark 6:5, NLT). I can see no reason why we should expect anything different. We should surely pray for such a day of His power. I wish to bear witness to God's readiness to answer prayer. Let us never grow tired of such an awesome privilege. May God also grant that we are entering a day of His power that will not only change lives but transform the church and the nation. In such a time we will surely see more of that healing grace in response to our prayers. In the meantime, let us rejoice in the healings we do see, seek to expand the ministry of healing and deepen our relationship with God.

Even so, come, Lord Jesus.

Chapter 8

NEW SONGS DISCOVERED IN THE NIGHT

Some Lessons from The Night School

It was a hot sunny day and the teacher was failing to grip the attention of her young pupils. Somehow the niceties of French irregular verbs seemed less appealing than being out in the sun and taking a dip in the cool river. It flowed tantalisingly close, just beyond their playing fields. As they dreamily gazed out of the windows, the green of the grass looked inviting. When anyone dared to let their eyes look away from the teacher long enough, they could just glimpse the glitter of the sun-kissed water of the river. As the teacher called for attention, did she remember her own childhood and what it was like to be a pupil shut in a classroom on a glorious day?

Lessons are hard to learn and often soon forgotten – especially, it seems, the lessons of life. I fear now that I have heard so much teaching, I am so much 'improved' by this teaching, that I am all too easily distracted. Old delights and new pleasures are now open to me. Like the schoolboy on a sunny day, I gaze with wonder at that which God has done; except now, as an adult, I have the freedom to walk out into the sunshine. Similarly, as those who have experienced the warmth and freedom of Christ's love, we can also know fullness of life through Him. We do, however, need to walk, or maybe with childlike enthusiasm, dance into it.

Perhaps it is time to pause and reflect on a few of the things I have learnt during illness and the time I returned to better health.

I have already touched on the issue of faith. In the trial itself my faith was that God would not only see me through, but somehow glorify His name. I had no assurance in the early part of my years of illness that I would be healed. There came a time of adjustment and then a kind of resignation to the realities of my condition. However, I began to find that challenged by my faith in God. I came to feel I should not passively slide into the clutches of the disease. I came to realise that there was a right kind of acceptance of what the disease was doing to me and there was a wrong kind of 'giving in' to its hold over my life. It could be compared to falling into a fast-flowing river. To resign yourself to the river and just let it carry you away and drag you under would be fatal. (Neither is it any use pretending you haven't fallen in!) Nor would it help to struggle in panic. The best policy is a calm assurance while battling to keep your head out of water often enough to breathe, and all the while making a determined attempt to swim to the riverbank. Similarly, there came a point when I had to energetically resist the symptoms of the disease. I did not note a date in my diary but the conviction grew that I should fight this ailment with whatever weapons I could find. It was not to be in angry panic, but in the same calm assurance of Christ's loving presence and strength. Then, unexpectedly one day, a gentle confidence was planted deep within me that I would be healed. It happened as I waited to see my specialist for a routine outpatient's appointment. As I observed fellow sufferers in more advanced stages of the disease it seemed that God said: 'That is not your future. You do not belong here.' It is hard to know at times whether you are hearing God or your own wishful thinking. But from time to time this confidence was underlined, including in a hotel room in

Vancouver. On the last day of my round the world trip on 25 November 2003, I had a sense I would be healed. But neither was I given a date in my diary, 'This is the day the Lord will take this from you.' This is no different from many Christians who have to 'wait for the Lord' to answer some prayer or promise. God has His own agenda and we can only submit to it. We can be confident that His time will be the right time. When we are able at last to see it all worked out in the realities of life it is wonderful.

I had no way of knowing what would happen between the 'promise' to be healed and the event taking place. For example, it could have been God's desire to bring me into a different kind of ministry first. So, when my health deteriorated in early 2004, I was uncertain where God was leading. It often seems God intervenes at the last minute and, if not the last minute for me exactly, it felt pretty close to it.

Reviewing that time of ill-health, enduring lessons are impressed upon me. For example, health and fitness are gifts from God to be valued and used for what is good and lasts. A colleague said to me, 'I must get more exercise'. This was in response to hearing of my routine of daily walking. After my healing I began to lose weight and rebuild my fitness levels. I did this by taking some simple and elementary care over what I ate and building into my daily 'programme' a few miles of walking. Responding to my friend, I said, 'The trouble is, you take your good health for granted.' Perhaps we all do until we lose it. I discovered what a privilege health and strength is – a blessing to be used and not abused. Abuse I would deem as not building a healthy lifestyle, and using up your time of good health on worthless things. None of us can know how long that period is. Serious illness can strike at any time and anybody. We assume when we are bounding around in youthful vigour that disability will not affect ourselves. Furthermore, for all of us the ageing process creeps up on us at an alarming rate. When I was at my worst, I would watch fit and able young people taking up habits of life that destroyed their health and ate up that available time. I wanted to shout out: 'Don't waste it!' Yet I knew that so often they were not in a position to hear. The lesson I constantly repeated to myself was, 'I know I have this moment in which to serve God or do this or that.' This meant learning to take opportunities as they presented themselves and not putting things off to another indefinite time in the future.

I have already said that I wonder whether we would have made the world trip had I not been ill. Not all issues were that dramatic. Day-to-day decisions were included. 'Live and serve Christ while you can,' was etched into my soul. The urgency and power of this, I believe, should not be lost. **This includes trusting God for now, not just for something that will happen in the future. It also means finding God's presence today** and seeking to serve Him today, not 'one day'. One day may never happen; **only now is certain** as far as this life is concerned. As a hospital chaplain, I used to hear patients who were newly retired say, 'We were so looking forward to retirement and this happens.' 'This' was some serious and life-threatening or permanent ailment. They would tell me how hard they had worked and saved and sacrificed for their comfortable dream of 'golden years' to come. How sad it is not to enjoy or be truly enriched by the journey of life itself. The advent of illness speaks of the value of learning to live in the joy and life of God now. Tomorrow will then look after itself. **The richer our experience of God now, the greater is our hope for tomorrow**. After all, it is Jesus we expect to meet in the events of the next day. The better we know Him, the more enchanting the prospect and the more wonderful heaven will seem to us, for **Jesus makes heaven heavenly.**

It is common experience that when life-threatening illness or long-lasting disability strikes, we assess our lives and ask the question: 'What is important?' Our relationship with God, certainly for the Christian, comes to the fore. I do not think it is God's way of getting our attention, but I do think that we are enabled to pay closer attention to God's voice and His priorities. Philip Yancey likens it to a hearing aid: 'When suffering strikes, it gives us the afflicted ones opportunity to turn up the volume and attend to a crucial message that we might otherwise ignore.' When I was ill, to serve at all often meant having to depend on God to give physical strength, the required energy and ability. 'Parkinson slump' doesn't seem to follow a pattern. For all Parkinson sufferers it seems to characteristically occur randomly. I would, for example, wake up to a day where my body ached, energy seemed drained and the world was enveloped in a kind of fog. I didn't lose my Christian joy but it wasn't easy to think of moving from the settee at all that day. This could happen on a Sunday, for example, when I was expected to lead a service of worship or preach or both. How should I respond?

Firstly, I have found, when tempted into an unhealthy lifestyle, that the best course is to stubbornly do the opposite. If the disease makes you feel you want to avoid company, then seek company out. I almost invariably felt better for doing so. To understand this, it should be noted that people suffering this disease face two kinds of pressure to keep away from other people, especially in public. One is the feeling of embarrassment as ability and dignity are taken away. Different people suffer different problems but slowness – like standing at the front of a queue whilst a line of impatient people wait for you to painstakingly try and find change to pay for a bill or shop purchases – clumsiness, drooling at the mouth, finishing food 15 minutes after everyone else, not being heard and therefore excluded in conversation, the fear of 'accident' because bladder or bowel control is difficult, are a few of those challenges. It can take courage to engage in simple socialising. Secondly, the sufferer on 'slump' days just doesn't feel up to it. Some Sundays I just felt, 'I can't do this today. I hurt too much and I don't feel able to raise the energy.' On such days I would ask Wendy to pray for me, add my bit and trust God to enable me to do what I had been called to. He never failed to provide the needed strength. I found that my physical need brought me into a new kind of dependence on God. Now my health is renewed, I pray that I remain dependent on God.

I have become utterly convinced that only God can effect real change in a person and draw someone into a dynamic relationship with Himself. In the same way only God can truly build the church. Although many would subscribe to that in theory, do we really believe it in practice? Certainly, I for one had some years of painful divine tuition before I truly recognised that methods, personal ability or training are not enough for Christian ministry. **The journey with God has been one of going down in my own ego and up in my admiration of Jesus and what He will do.** It was a long time before I made prayer not **a** priority of ministry but **the** priority. I have met colleagues who admit to being mighty busy but have a minimal prayer commitment. Part of the advantage of restored health is being able to renew old habits of prayer out of a new dimension of dependence drawn from my time of ill-health. My testimony is to a heavenly Father Who strengthened and enabled me in the trial of the illness as well as delivered me from many of its symptoms. I readily identify with Daniel's three friends Shadrach, Meshach and Abednego, who faced the fury of the tyrant King Nebuchadnezzar. When commanded to bow down in worship before the King's imposing image, they alone refused. The account records:

'Then Nebuchadnezzar flew into a rage and ordered Shadrach, Meshach, and Abednego to be brought before him. When they were brought in, Nebuchadnezzar said to them, "Is it true, Shadrach, Meshach, and Abednego, that you refuse to serve my gods or to worship the gold statue I have set up? I will give you one more chance. If you bow down and worship the statue I have made when you hear the sound of the musical instruments, all will be well. But if you refuse, you will be thrown immediately into the blazing furnace. What god will be able to rescue you from my power then?" Shadrach,

Meshach, and Abednego replied, "O Nebuchadnezzar, we do not need to defend ourselves before you. If we are thrown into the blazing furnace, the God whom we serve is able to save us. He will rescue us from your power, Your Majesty. But even if he doesn't, Your Majesty can be sure that we will never serve your gods or worship the gold statue you have set up.'" (Daniel 3:13-18, NLT.) *

If my experience was nothing to do with tyrants and furnaces, my response, I was convinced, should be similar. My God was able to heal but even if He did not I would serve Him. The outcome was similar too. Having had the three flung into the furnace, Nebuchadnezzar sat down to watch their death throes:

'But suddenly, as he was watching, Nebuchadnezzar jumped up in amazement and exclaimed to his advisers, "Didn't we tie up three men and throw them into the furnace?" "Yes," they said, "we did indeed, Your Majesty." "Look!" Nebuchadnezzar shouted. "I see four men, unbound, walking around in the fire. They aren't even hurt by the flames! And the fourth looks like a divine being!" Then Nebuchadnezzar came as close as he could to the door of the flaming furnace and shouted: "Shadrach, Meshach, and Abednego, servants of the Most High God, come out! Come here!" So Shadrach, Meshach, and Abednego stepped out of the fire.' (Daniel 3:24-26, NLT.)

My Lord was indeed with me in the trial and brought me out of it. How can I doubt Him now? May I never outlive my faith or love of Him.

I made note earlier of how much sharper and more precious the glimpses of the world and life seemed

---

* *Holy Bible: New Living Translation.* 1997. Wheaton, Ill.: Tyndale House.

when in the grip of Parkinson's disease. When I was not sure how much longer I would be able to enjoy them, they seemed dressed in brighter colours. My return to health brought with it a pain-free opportunity to experience and savour things once denied me or restricted. The sheer elation at being able to taste and smell things again, to walk freely, remains hard to describe. I began to appreciate the blessings of the ordinary. To have an 'ordinary' day again was to me extra-ordinary. To stir in the morning from sleep, turn over pain-free, luxuriate in the soft sheets and drift off to sleep again, was an exultant joy. Such simple delights had me nearly dancing in praise to God next day. Not surprisingly, each day was filled with such delights. I am still dismayed it took such an illness to bring me to properly appreciate the wonder of every-day things. Perhaps if I had learnt to savour life and not rush so madly through it, to take notice of things, even the movements of my own body, and thank God for them all, I would have seen this more clearly earlier in my life. Here, then, is today's task too. In all this, **it is possible to revel in what is good or to descend into misery**. We can make that choice. We can accept what is good in our lives and be thankful and rejoice in them, or we can moan into misery. Victor Frankel says: 'Despair is suffering without meaning, and everything can be taken from a man but one thing: the last of the human freedoms – to choose one's attitude in any given set of circumstances.'

All of these things emphasise to me the astonishing magnitude of God's grace. Grace means that I receive what I don't deserve. My healing, the ability to live and serve God and others, the weight of everyday blessings I have just mentioned and above all the gift of eternal life and all that is included with that are piled upon me. In listing these things I have hardly even begun to name the range of good things God has given me, and all this despite my many failures and weaknesses. I am massively in debt to a wonderful heavenly Father and can never thank Him enough or give Him enough. That is the way it is with God – He loves to give fools like me a new life and enrich that life with the things that count. As this account I hope demonstrates, the path is not always easy, but it is good. There are plenty of surprises, too: not all pleasant ones, but the long-term outcomes are amazing. The call is to keep true to Him in the faith that He will fulfil His good purpose and will not fail us. The sadness in all this is that so many fail to respond to His invitation to receive what He is so ready to give.

When all things are considered I am simply outclassed when it comes to generosity and giving by a loving heavenly Father.

Out given

Gifts come in all kinds of packages
Some gaudy and overstated, pretending,
And far outclassing
That which they conceal.
Others plain and ordinary
Seem to tell another story
And little promising
The treasure it will reveal.
Gifts are given with all kinds of attitudes
Some dutiful and obligated, hoping
To satisfy some demand
That burdens the reluctant giver.
Some bear a weight of meaning
Carrying the freight of caring
To express true devotion
Of a kind that can never find full expression.

Gifts have different kinds of value.
Some that cost little to the giver
Seem generous to the receiver
And are prized beyond expectation.
Others that were bought taking great pain

Are hardly opened and lain
To one side, are dismissed thoughtlessly
And thrown into a corner carelessly.

But the greatest gifts by far
Cannot be found in catalogues or shops
Nor advertised by TV star,
And bought by card or cash.
But the best and highest giving
Is an act of loving, spending
A life of selfless caring for another.
Most extravagant of all is in sacrificing
Your life for sister or brother.

Before this all other presents seem small
And me, the amazed receiver of it all,
My health and life and joy and peace,
Can only wonder
But can never
Return gratitude, and as myself the giver,
Nor can I adequately match
This matchless gift of Yours
But simply bow with worship that adores.

Chapter 9

SONGS THAT WERE HEARD IN THE NIGHT

Still Learning

In fighting to survive the dark nights, the light shines not just in the struggle itself but at various occasions during the rest of life. Perhaps new depth or some modification of our understanding of life is necessary, or total rejection is needed. Are our beliefs and understanding of life ever totally static? Anyway, what follows are further reflections drawn my own experience and that of others whom I have sought to support. It remains true, I believe, that we either grow in our relationship with God, led by Jesus and enabled by the Holy Spirit, or we go backwards. We can find ourselves getting more critical, less engaged: with worship, other people's service, Christian teaching, and a world of many miseries. When such a jaundiced response settles upon our souls, we tend to think that we have, in various degrees, lost faith. Yet I wonder whether it is always so. Sometimes, is it the rebellious reaction to God in action that is a personal protest at having to go through 'all of this'?

All the time, God has two arms stretched out to hold you before you drown in the pool of tears. God doesn't blame anyone for tears, but He wants to advance us in His Kingdom and mission. In the threatening darkness He gives strength and courage.

In 2005, I attended the meetings of the World Baptist Alliance in Birmingham, UK. I walked past a man several times who stood next to a stall touting for support for some charity or other. Resplendent in his dog collar that announced his status (!) he shouted, 'Cheer up, it may never happen.' As mentioned elsewhere, it is a common feature of Parkinson's for the face to be 'frozen' with an unsunny look. I did not comment at the time, but I did wonder what he hoped to gain by such a remark. It happens I was feeling joyous, not gloomy. He was at the very least guilty of judging by appearances, always a hazardous occupation. Further, any chance he might have had of bringing some blessing to me was blown out of the water by one silly comment. Again, there was no thought of discovering if I did have a major issue. Perhaps the real problem is a lack of love – do we care for each other if it costs us empathy, time and endurance?

I have mentioned that for any one of us, throughout life, this **starts with our relationship with God,** for that will determine everything else. Prayer is an important component of this. I made what I consider to be a major step forward when I made prayer the priority of ministry. My poem at the end of the chapter reflects this. Like archaeologists who scrape away the dirt and grime that have obscured ancient artefacts from view, so God uncovers the person we are meant to be. We are not static, like a statue turned out of a mould and set up in a public square. That sculpture, however well crafted, is going nowhere. We are going somewhere. By serving ourselves, we live in the tiny space of our own corrupted desires. As we hammer it into our preferred shape, the more it turns ugly in our hands. On the other hand, if we pursue '*love, joy, peace, patience, kindliness, self-control*' (Galatians 5:22) and similar qualities, with the help of God's Holy Spirit we are shaped, piece by piece, into the people God intended us to be. He would make us somewhat reminiscent of Jesus, but dressed in *our* clothes, working in *our* workplaces. This is possible even if, like me, you face restrictions. Is this real? Does trusting God make any difference? Certainly, for me it has made a massive difference. I still have a purpose, a hope, an inner strength, joy, and love mediated through family and my church. Followers of Christ find, for example, that hope beckons us onwards whatever the situation.

With hope therefore, I continued to minister, at first continuing in London, although it was a struggle. The Christian church has a very high calling to represent Christ to the world, in both our individual and our corporate lives. It is no easy task to become this very special community as it is counter-cultural. Usually, when that transformative relationship with God grows, our prayer life develops too. Prayer is, after all, a conversation with our heavenly Father. Ideally, all aspects of His character, His nature and His deeds inform our prayers. In that sense, it is far more than a conversation: it is a response to the glory and wonder of God as He comes close to us. As a minister it was my habit to pray for every member of my church regularly and often, as well as a variety of other issues. You may think that means that my prayers were request-dominated. This would be far from the truth. I would frequently find myself overwhelmed by God's presence.

My ailment has brought a challenge to this. Although I think I have made progress, I have yet to fully resolve this issue. The problems that Parkinson's creates for the would-be pray-er are a shortage of energy, concentration, and endurance. Our prayers need all these and more. If we struggle against this, the more the body protests. In trying to overcome this, I recognised the need for prayer to be **habitual** and **continual**. By this I mean:

Habitual – that we have a fixed time each day for devotions which acts as a launchpad to living the rest of the day with God. We develop habits to build the structure of our lives. When we make prayer a key part of that, we can place Christ at the centre of our activities.

Continual – By continual I mean continuing the life of prayer through our waking hours.

I maintain these two aspects of prayer; I have tried to enhance continuing prayer but have not done as well with it as I had hoped. This dual aspect for prayer remains my preferred solution in my circumstances. I mention all this in the hope it will help someone. I am not claiming to be some kind of prayer expert, but because I have benefited in the past from mature followers of Christ when they explained their practice of prayer. Perhaps it would be far better to check the Bible characters like Moses, Daniel and Nehemiah. Supremely it is Jesus Himself who shows us the way. Yet those who have physical limitations must battle all the more fiercely to ensure that physical disability doesn't bring us spiritual decline. Praise God that Jesus' resurrection power enables to stand up against the onslaught and win.

It is not only spiritual exercises in which we are given help – it is physical exercise too. In 2002, whilst I hadn't quite seized up, we took the opportunity to attempt to walk the West Highland Way. This challenging track is 96 miles long from Glasgow to Fort William. We attempted this with our two good friends, Kerry and Nancy from Australia, eighteen months after diagnosis. **This is another example of taking opportunities when they turn up**. How, then, did I get on walking not just one day, but day after day? I quote various extracts from a light-hearted account I wrote at the time. Several days into the sodden and somewhat muddy walk I noted that:

> '*Something should be done about gaiters. We often resorted to helping each other in the struggle, me in particular sought help from Wendy. Another indication of lost ability. Walking stick, grey beard, thinning hair, creaking legs, slowness, clumsiness, altogether not a vision of youthful vigour.*'

Later on at Doune Bothy:*

'After a time I thought I should drink some coffee from the flask, and stood up to retrieve my pack. "All my legs ache," I said, memorably. Everyone, especially my companions, scrutinised me carefully in case they had missed a limb or two.'

Then on the last leg (!) of the last day:

'Feeling like doing nothing more than lying down and resting for a day and a half, I decided that the only thing was to bite the lip and place one foot in front of another in imitation of a squaddie. Footsore as I was, this may not have looked very impressive, but it got me there. I seem to remember whistling or something like that as well. Think, therefore, of an overweight man with thin hair, grey beard, pack on back, walking like a geriatric walrus whilst whistling breathlessly and badly, and you will catch a glimpse of just what a heroic figure I cut. How long can a mile be? This one seemed to stretch like a bungee rope. Then the sight all Way walkers look for – a car park. This is not because we wanted to hitch a lift, but because inside this car park was the goal of all our efforts. We plodded up to it and gathered round the sign that said 'The End of the West Highland Way' like worshippers at a wayside shrine. The elation was vast. I had done it. After the diagnosis and the growing sense of incapacity I had yet managed this. It was a blow against my foe, even though a very painful one at times, and I was triumphant.'

This is a reminder there are often still good things to experience even if tougher than we expect. It would be wrong of me if I give the impression that every day was an

---

* A bothy is a kind of shelter equipped with fireplace and sleeping shelf and nothing else.

exercise in endurance against pain. Some days I felt close to what I was before Parkinson's. Yet such days never announced themselves beforehand. So planning ahead became hazardous at best.

When talking about faith, our hope spurs us on through everything. Imagine then that moment when we exchange this life for the next, meet Jesus with love in His eyes – the love that scarred His body and saved us. Then we will be able to shout, 'I have made it, for He has brought me through', and join the exultant worshippers.

The unhurried place

Find the unhurried space,
The place where, without haste,
You draw aside
Alone,
But not alone.

Find the still place,
That hush
Which steals like
An evening shadow
Across
The troubled soul.

Find the peaceful place,
That spot,
That shelter fashioned
By irresistible command
For calm
Where He masters the storm.

Find the quiet space,
The pause
Where open ears,
Deaf to demands,

SONGS THAT WERE HEARD IN THE NIGHT

Hear
The gentle whisper of His voice.

Find the meeting place,
Just you and Him together.
Contrive no agenda,
Target no self-achievement
Except
The companionship of friends.

Find the healing grace
That comes to end the haemorrhage of life
With the accumulated wounds
Of strife.
Stretch there a hand.
Touch, and be touched again.

Seek to see the face
That smiles
With delight in you.
Waste time with Him
For wasting time is not wasted
With Him,
Bearing fruit in all the hurrying
Hours.

Find the unhurried place,
The space
Where the Creator
Re-creates and shapes,
And with intent
Hand-crafts
Your clay to love's
Embodiment.

Walk with unhurried pace
With Him.
Tread busy streets

In cloistered calm.
Bring peace
To peaceless people with no
Place.

God said: 'There is a place near me.' Exodus.33:21

Chapter 10

SONGS THAT STILL RING IN HEART AND SOUL

Update & Footnotes in Later Years

It was an amazing day that March afternoon as I watched people crowd into the chapel to mark the end of my service as Baptist pastor.

'Do you think you are healed forever?' I was asked soon after I first testified to my restoration. This is not an unreasonable question to ask about a progressive disease. My answer is still relevant: 'I know what God has done now. I cannot predict the future.'

As I reflect on my healing 19 years after diagnosis, I know that the condition has deteriorated to some extent in retirement. However, my condition treats me to different symptoms than it did in those first three years. But I received from God what was needed to sustain and enable me to complete the course until I reached normal retirement age. Furthermore, those years were not unproductive years, but God used me during that time. I am so grateful to Him for this kindness. To me, retirement day was like crossing the line at the end of a long-distance race. There was a sense of elation, but at the same time relief that I could rest for a while. Some predicted I would never retire, but I feel God made sure I did. However, there is always the opportunity to minister the love of Christ even if roles change. At the moment my physical condition limits my activities and it is difficult to define what kind of a ministry I now have. So I try and concentrate on being Christ's kind of person, encouraging where I can and serving when able to do so. Increasingly, writing has seemed to be a calling too. This too has its challenges as do most activities of life.

One such challenge involved something I have alluded to but not enlarged upon. Suffice it to say that on one recent occasion I was admitted to hospital for a minor procedure. The problem was brought about by an extremely painful twisted bowel. I was not treated for some six hours or so. As I waited, I swelled like a balloon and when, eventually, I had relief I deflated like a balloon as well. Some weeks later I was invited in for surgery (after a repeat performance on my part) and as I was wheeled into the operating theatre was asked: 'What do you do?' 'I am retired,' I informed my questioner. His reply: 'What do you do now you are retired?' – for all the world as if I was a contestant in game show and not surrounded by surgeons and nurses together with an anaesthetist poised and ready to deliver the knock-out blow. Considering the occasion, I merely said: 'Surviving'.

My story has inevitably raised questions of healing and I have tried to incorporate some thoughts on this, and on my experience, enriched by my involvement with the suffering and reflections of others. The world I have been surrounded by tends, when it thinks of healing, to have a mind governed by the idea that the body is essentially a kind of machine. So, to heal is to mend the machine, if possible, back to working order. The healer we would then make to be some kind of high-order mechanic. What is more, increasingly, diagnostic machines are being developed and used to treat medical conditions. Just like a modern car, I will soon just hook up to a computer and it will tell me what is wrong and order the necessary treatment. Maybe, like supermarkets and libraries, we won't need to see a doctor but just go online and the medical supercomputer will do all that's necessary! But such a scheme would be essentially mechanistic – material cause and effect in a world governed by fixed laws. So, what works today will work tomorrow, if genuine. For example, 'cold fusion'* was said to be demonstrated by a particular set of experiments, but when found to be unrepeatable, the theory lost credibility. Outcomes have then to be predictable and follow 'fixed' laws to be accepted by orthodox science. Newton, and many like him since, have seen their explorations as discovering the mind of God as they observed the natural forces of the universe. But recent science toys with less neat theories, for example, Heisenberg's uncertainty principle – well, not so recent as all that! – and chaos theory.

In looking at claims for divine healing, many are basically sceptical, not having personally witnessed such a healing and hearing of people who seem to have become wealthy because of their 'healing ministry' gives them reasons. There are Christians today who concede this, though many do not. They believe that in the early days of the church, God gave His people miraculous powers to confirm that the message of Jesus was not some wild fantasy. They believe that once the Bible was recognised by the church as God's inspired message, miracles were no longer necessary since the Bible contained all that was needed for life and godliness. Whilst this may be true of the Bible as 'God's word,' Christ's compassion is intended to be portrayed in the lives of His people. So, why did a large part of the church move away from this ministry? True compassion would demand the use of any effective means to relieve the sufferer. Christ's compassion is surely the same as it ever was. It would seem, therefore, that He would desire His servants to be actively involved in battling against the misery-creating bodily misfunctions.

---

* That is, nuclear fusion at a manageably low temperature, rather than the 'hot fusion' that naturally occurs in stars and our own sun at many millions of degrees Celsius.

It is no surprise that the gospels record that Jesus included healing the sick as part of the church's ministry.

By the Reformation, this call to respond to the needy world had become a cynical exploitation of the poor and ignorant, claiming a bit of wood was a piece of 'the true cross' or a fragment of bone once belonged to a famous martyr. Where many today raise funds through raffles or sponsored runs, they had relics. These 'relics' were sold as having miraculous powers. The superstitions of the gullible enabled unscrupulous men to use them as a promotional tool and as propaganda. 'Come touch the bones of St Thomas à Becket. Many have been healed. Even the King who had him murdered had to kneel at his casket.' Crowds have been travelling to Canterbury ever since Becket was murdered in 1170. Those seriously ill or maimed became targets then and now. All this was far from the spirit of Jesus, and the reformers were eager to say so. Healing by God or some object sanctioned by the 'church' fell increasingly into disrepute. It seemed to be the province of charlatans and con men. Did the reformers, in their eagerness to be rid of such things, go too far?

When it comes to healing today, I believe we would do well to avoid the flamboyant 'acts' who appear on stage more like showmen. Frequently advertised with sensationalist claims ('See wheelchairs thrown away', etc.), they seem to ape some sort of grand magician. Surely our desire is to follow Jesus' lead. He simply and quietly met the sufferer's need, whatever it was, individual by individual. Shouldn't we as His representatives simply in His name seek to do the same? Each person needs to be heard and then we should seek to lead them into the love of God.

In Him we find our purpose, our prospects and our peace with God, with others and with ourselves. A lady once told me after I had been restored: 'Now you have a testimony' – not that I didn't have one before, but now it was something special. Well, I do have a testimony. It is to God who radically directed my path through life. He has strengthened me, inspired me, shaped me, healed me in different ways and always granted me His joy, His peace, and His astonishing love. I have found it to be extra-ordinary in its dimensions, its reach, its endeavour, its courage, its gentle triumph. However, it is no 'it' that has mesmerised me for nearly all my life. It is Jesus. That remains true.

To God be all the glory.

Secret strength

How can we stand in days of trial?
When the storms gather, and sorrow abounds?
When agendas grow long and demands increase
Our energies waste, and there's no time for ease,
Where is the means to more than survive,
And in joyous freedom to revive?

You are our secret strength
The rock of our defence
Our hope beyond despair.
You are the shelter in the storm,
The shade against the burning sun,
You are life indestructible
And love inexhaustible,
You are the one with wisdom and insight
To turn us from darkness to enter the light.

We come then to You, Jesus our Lord,
Of every good thing the source,
In time of need the resource,
For You are our secret strength,
Who, in love turns weakness into might.
Let us stand, then, for what is right.
Trust Him however dark the night
To bring us through into love's light.
So let songs resound throughout the night
In hope, and joy, and hearts at peace.